Current Clinical Strategies

Surgery

Sixth Edition

The University of California, Irvine, Manual of Surgery

Samuel Eric Wilson, MD
Professor and Chairman
Department of Surgery
College of Medicine
University of California, Irvine

Bruce M. Achauer, MD
John A. Butler, MD
David A. Chamberlin, MD
Paul D. Chan, MD
Marianne Cinat, MD
Roger Crumley, MD
Alex Di Stante, MD
C. Garo Gholdoian, MD
Ian L. Gordon, MD, PhD
Joshua Helman, MD
James G. Jakowatz, MD
Fernando Kafie, MD
Michael E. Lekawa, MD
I. James Sarfeh, MD
Michelle Schultz, MD
Harry Skinner, MD
Charles Theuer, MD
Russell A. Williams, MD

Current Clinical Strategies Publishing

www.ccspublishing.com/ccs

Digital Book and Updates

Purchasers of this book may download the digital book and updates for Palm, Pocket PC, Windows and Macintosh. The digital books can be downloaded at the Current Clinical Strategies Publishing Internet site:

www.ccspublishing.com/ccs/surg.htm

Copyright © 2006 Current Clinical Strategies Publishing. All rights reserved. This book, or any parts thereof, may not be reproduced, photocopied, or stored in an information retrieval network without the permission of the publisher. The reader is advised to consult the drug package insert and other references before using any therapeutic agent. The publisher disclaims any liability, loss, injury, or damage incurred as a consequence, directly or indirectly, of the use and application of any of the contents of this text.

Current Clinical Strategies Publishing
27071 Cabot Road
Laguna Hills, California 92653
Phone: 800-331-8227 or 949-348-8404
Internet: www.ccspublishing.com/ccs
E-mail: info@ccspublishing.com

Printed in USA

ISBN 1929622-57-0

Table of Contents

Surgical Documentation 5
   Surgical History and Physical Examination 5
   Preoperative Preparation of the Surgical Patient 6
   Admitting and Preoperative Orders 7
   Preoperative Note 8
   Brief Operative Note 8
   Operative Report 8
   Postoperative Check 9
   Postoperative Orders 10
   Postoperative Surgical Management 10
   Surgical Progress Note 11
   Procedure Note 12
   Discharge Note 12
   Discharge Summary 13
   Prescription Writing 13

Clinical Care of the Surgical Patient 14
   Radiographic Evaluation of Common Interventions 14
   Blood Component Therapy 15
   Fluids and Electrolytes 16
   Evaluation of Postoperative Fever 16
   Sepsis 17
   Nutrition in the Surgical Patient 23
   Total Parental Nutrition 24
   Central Venous Catheterization 27
   Pulmonary Artery Catheterization 29
   Normal Pulmonary Artery Catheter Values 29
   Venous Cutdown 30
   Arterial Line Placement 30
   Cricothyrotomy 31

Trauma 32
   Management of the Trauma Patient 32
   Penetrating Abdominal Trauma 33
   Blunt Abdominal Trauma 34
   Head Trauma 35
   Thoracic Trauma 37
   Tension Pneumothorax 38
   Flail Chest 38
   Massive Hemothorax 38
   Cardiac Tamponade 39
   Other Life-Threatening Trauma Emergencies 40
   Burns 41

Pulmonary Disorders 45
   Airway Management and Intubation 45
   Ventilator Management 46
   Epistaxis 47

Disorders of the Alimentary Tract 51
   Acute Abdomen 51
   Appendicitis 54
   Appendectomy 55

Hernias	57
Inguinal Hernia Repair Technique	59
Upper Gastrointestinal Bleeding	61
Esophageal Varices	63
Helicobacter Pylori Infection and Peptic Ulcer Disease	65
Lower Gastrointestinal Bleeding	70
Anorectal Disorders	74
Hemorrhoids	74
Anal fissures	75
Levator ani syndrome and proctalgia fugax	75
Pruritus ani	76
Perianal abscess	76
Fistula-in-Ano	77
Colorectal Cancer	77
Mesenteric Ischemia	80
Intestinal Obstruction	81
Acute Pancreatitis	83
Acute Cholecystitis	86
Laparoscopic Cholecystectomy Procedure	87
Open Cholecystectomy Procedure	89
Choledocholithiasis	90

Disorders of the Breast 91
   Breast Cancer Screening and Diagnosis 91
   Breast Cysts 93
   Fibroadenomas 94
   Breast Cancer 94

Urologic Disorders 97
   Prostate Cancer 97
   Renal Colic 101
   Urologic Emergencies 103
      Acute urinary retention 103
      Testicular torsion 104
      Priapism 105

Vascular and Orthopedic Surgery 106
   Peripheral Arterial Occlusive Disease 106
   Abdominal Aortic Aneurysms 108
   Orthopedic Fractures and Dislocations 109
   Ankle Sprains 112

Index 114

/ Surgical History and Physical Examination 5

Surgical Documentation

S. E. Wilson, MD

Surgical History and Physical Examination

Identifying Data: Patient's name, age, race, sex; referring physician.
Chief Compliant: Reason given by patient for seeking surgical care and the duration of the symptom.
History of Present Illness (HPI): Describe the course of the patient's illness, including when it began, character of the symptoms; pain onset (gradual or rapid), precise character of pain (constant, intermittent, cramping, stabbing, radiating); other factors associated with pain (defecation, urination, eating, strenuous activities); location where the symptoms began; aggravating or relieving factors. Vomiting (color, character, blood, coffee-ground emesis, frequency, associated pain). Change in bowel habits; rectal bleeding, character of blood (clots, bright or dark red), trauma; recent weight loss or anorexia; other related diseases; past diagnostic testing.
Past Medical History (PMH): Previous operations and indications; dates and types of procedures; serious injuries, hospitalizations; diabetes, hypertension, peptic ulcer disease, asthma, heart disease; hernia, gallstones.
Medications: Aspirin, anticoagulants, hypertensive and cardiac medications, diuretics.
Allergies: Penicillin, codeine, iodine.
Family History: Medical problems in relatives. Family history of colon cancer, cardiovascular disease.
Social History: Alcohol, smoking, drug usage, occupation, daily activity. *hand dominance*
Review of Systems (ROS):
  General: Weight gain or loss; loss of appetite, fever, fatigue, night sweats. Activity level.
  HEENT: Headaches, seizures, sore throat, masses, dentures.
  Respiratory: Cough, sputum, hemoptysis, dyspnea on exertion, ability to walk up flight of stairs.
  Cardiovascular: Chest pain, orthopnea, claudication, extremity edema.
  Gastrointestinal: Dysphagia, vomiting, abdominal pain, hematemesis, melena (black tarry stools), hematochezia (bright red blood per rectum), constipation, change in bowel habits; hernia, hemorrhoids, gallstones.
  Genitourinary: Dysuria, hesitancy, hematuria, discharge; impotence, prostate problems, urinary frequency.
  Gynecological: Last menstrual period, gravida, para, abortions, length of regular cycle and periods, birth control.
  Skin: Easy bruising, bleeding tendencies.
  Neurological: Stroke, transient ischemic attacks, weakness, *numbness, tingling*

Surgical Physical Examination
General appearance: Note whether the patient looks "ill," well, or malnourished.
Vital Signs: Temperature, respirations, heart rate, blood pressure, weight.
Eyes: Pupils equally round and react to light (PERRL); extraocular movements intact (EOMI).
Neck: Jugular venous distention (JVD), thyromegaly, masses, bruits; lymphadenopathy; trachea midline.

6 Preoperative Preparation of the Surgical Patient

Chest: Equal expansion, dullness to percussion; rales, rhonchi, breath sounds.
Heart: Regular rate and rhythm (RRR), first and second heart sounds; murmurs (grade 1-6), pulses (graded 0-2+).
Breast: Skin retractions, erythema, tenderness, masses (mobile, fixed), nipple discharge, axillary or supraclavicular node enlargement.
Abdomen: Contour (flat, scaphoid, obese, distended), scars, bowel sounds, bruits, tenderness, masses, liver span; splenomegaly, guarding, rebound, percussion note (dull, tympanic), pulsatile masses, costovertebral angle tenderness (CVAT), abdominal hernias.
Genitourinary: Inguinal hernias, testicles, varicoceles; urethral discharge, varicocele.
Extremities: Skin condition, edema (grade 1-4+); cyanosis, clubbing, pulses (radial, ulnar, femoral, popliteal, posterior tibial, dorsalis pedis; simultaneous palpation of radial and femoral pulses). Grading of pulses: 0 = absent; 1+ weak; 2+ normal; 3+ very strong (arterial dilation).
Rectal Exam: Masses, tenderness, hemorrhoids, prostate masses; bimanual palpation, guaiac test for occult blood.
Neurological: Mental status, cranial nerves, gait, strength (graded 0-5); tendon reflexes, sensory testing.
Laboratory Evaluation: Electrolytes (sodium, potassium, bicarbonate, chloride, BUN, creatinine), glucose, liver function tests, INR/PTT, CBC with differential; X-rays, ECG (if older than 35 yrs or cardiovascular disease), urine analysis.
Assessment (Impression): Assign a number to each problem and discuss each problem. Begin with most important problem and rank in order.
Plan: Discuss surgical plans for each numbered problem, including preoperative testing, laboratory studies, medications, antibiotics, endoscopy.

Preoperative Preparation of the Surgical Patient

1. Review the patient's history and physical examination, and write a preoperative note assessing the patient's overall condition and operative risk.
2. **Preoperative laboratory evaluation:** Electrolytes, BUN, creatinine, INR/PTT, CBC, platelet count, UA, ABG, pulmonary function test. Chest x-ray (>35 yrs old), EKG (if older then 35 yrs old or if cardiovascular disease). Type and cross for an appropriate number of units of blood. No screening laboratory tests are required in the healthy patient.
3. **Skin preparation:** Patient to shower and scrub the operative site with germicidal soap (Hibiclens) on the night before surgery. On the day of surgery, hair should be removed with an electric clipper or shaved just prior to operation.
4. **Prophylactic antibiotics or endocarditis prophylaxis** if indicated.
5. **Preoperative incentive spirometry** on the evening prior to surgery may be indicated for patients with pulmonary disease.
6. **Thromboembolic** prophylaxis should be provided for selected, high-risk patients.
7. **Diet:** NPO after midnight. → no pressors! for flap patients
8. **IV and monitoring lines:** At least one 18-gauge IV for initiation of anesthesia. Arterial catheter and pulmonary artery catheters (Swan-Ganz) if indicated. Patient to void on call to operating room.
9. **Medications.** Preoperative sedation as ordered by anesthesiologist. Maintenance medications to be given the morning of surgery with a sip of water. Diabetics should receive one half of their usual AM insulin dose, and

an insulin drip should be initiated with hourly glucose monitoring. *Intraop?*

10. Bowel preparation

Bowel preparation is required for upper or lower GI tract procedures.

Antibiotic Preparation for Colonic Surgery

Mechanical Prep: Day 1: Clear liquid diet, laxative (milk of magnesia 30 cc or magnesium citrate 250 cc), tap water or Fleet enemas until clear. Day 2: Clear liquid diet, NPO, laxative. Day 3: Operation.

Whole Gut Lavage: Polyethylene glycol electrolyte solution (GoLytely). Day 1: 2 liters PO or per nasogastric tube over 5 hours. Clear liquid diet. Day 2: Operation.

Oral Antibiotic Prep: One day prior to surgery, after mechanical or whole gut lavage, give neomycin 1 gm and erythromycin 250 mg at 1 p.m., 2 p.m., 11 p.m.

11. Preoperative IV antibiotics: Initiate preoperatively and give one dose during operation and one dose of antibiotic postoperatively. Cefotetan (Cefotan), 1 gm IV q12h, for bowel flora, or cefazolin (Ancef), 1 gm IVPB q8h x 3 doses, for clean procedures.

12. Anticoagulants: Discontinue Coumadin 5 days preop and check PT; stop IV heparin 6 hours prior to surgery. *What about Lovenox?*

Admitting and Preoperative Orders

Admit to: Ward, ICU, or preoperative room.
Diagnosis: Intended operation and indication.
Condition: Stable
Vital Signs: Frequency of vital signs; input and output recording; neurological or vascular checks. Notify physician if blood pressure <90/60, >160/110; pulse >110; pulse <60; temperature >101.5; urine output <35 cc/h for >2 hours; respiratory rate >30.
Activity: Bed rest or ambulation; bathroom privileges.
Allergies: No known allergies
Diet: NPO (ADAT)
IV Orders: D5 1/2 NS at 100 cc/hour.
Oxygen: 6 L/min by nasal canula.
Drains: Foley catheter to closed drainage. Nasogastric tube at low intermittent suction. Other drains, tubes, dressing changes. Orders for irrigation of tubes.
Medications: Antibiotics to be initiated immediately preoperatively; additional dose during operation and 1 dose of antibiotic postoperatively. Cefotetan (Cefotan), 1 gm IV q12h, for bowel flora, or cefazolin (Ancef) 1 gm IVPB q8h x 3 doses;) for clean procedures.
Labs and Special X-Rays: Electrolytes, BUN, creatinine, INR/PTT, CBC, platelet count, UA, ABG, pulmonary function tests. Chest x-ray (if >35 yrs old), EKG (if older then 35 yrs old or if cardiovascular disease). Type and cross for an appropriate number of units of blood.

Preoperative Note

Preoperative Diagnosis:
Procedure Planned:
Type of Anesthesia Planned:
Laboratory Data: Electrolytes, BUN, creatinine, CBC, INR/PTT, UA, EKG, chest x-ray; type and screen for blood or cross match if indicated; liver function tests, ABG.
Risk Factors: Cardiovascular, pulmonary, hepatic, renal, coagulopathic, nutritional risk factors. *(heart dz, lung dz, liver dz, kidney dz, bleeding d/o)*
American Surgical Association (ASA) grading of surgical risk: 1= normal; 2= mild systemic disease; 3= severe systemic disease; 4= disease with major threat to life; 5= not expected to survive.
Consent: Document explanation to patient of risks and benefits of the procedure and alternative treatments. Document patient's or guardian's informed consent and understanding of the procedure. Obtain signed consent form.
Allergies:
Major Medical Problems:
Medications:
Special Requirements: Signed blood transfusion consent form; documentation that breast procedure patients have been given an information brochure.

Brief Operative Note

This note should be written in chart immediately after the surgical procedure.
Date of the Procedure:
Preoperative Diagnosis:
Postoperative Diagnosis:
Procedure:
Operative Findings:
Names of Surgeon and Assistants:
Anesthesia: General endotracheal, spinal, epidural, regional or local.
Estimated Blood Loss (EBL):
Fluids and Blood Products Administered During Procedure:
Urine output:
Specimens: Pathology specimens, cultures, blood samples.
Intraoperative X-rays:
Drains:
Condition of Patient: Stable

Operative Report

This full report should be dictated at the conclusion of the surgical procedure.
Identifying Data: Name of patient, medical record number; name of dictating physician, date of dictation.
Attending Surgeon and Service:
Date of Procedure:
Preoperative Diagnosis:
Postoperative Diagnosis:

Procedure Performed:
Names of Surgeon and Assistants:
Type of Anesthesia Used:
Estimated Blood Loss (EBL):
Fluid and Blood Products Administered During Operation:
Specimens: Pathology, cultures, blood samples.
Drains and Tubes Placed:
Complications:
Consultations Intraoperatively:
Indications for Surgery: Brief history of patient and indications for surgery.
Findings: Describe gross findings and frozen section results relayed to operating room.
Description of Operation: Position of patient; skin prep and draping; location and types of incisions; details of procedure from beginning to end, including description of surgical findings, both normal and abnormal. Intraoperative studies or x-rays; hemostatic and closure techniques; dressings applied. Needle and sponge counts as reported by operative nurse. Patient's condition and disposition. Send copies of report to surgeons and referring physicians.

Postoperative Check

A postoperative check should be completed on the evening after surgery. This check is similar to a daily progress note.

Example Postoperative Check

Date/time:
Postoperative Check
Subjective: Note any patient complaints, and note the adequacy of pain relief.
Objective:
  General appearance:
  Vitals: Maximum temperature in the last 24 hours (T_{max}), current temperature, pulse, respiratory rate, blood pressure.
  Urine Output: If urine output is less than 30 cc per hour, more fluids should be infused if the patient is hypovolemic.
  Physical Exam:
  Chest and lungs:
  Abdomen:
  Wound Examination: The wound should be examined for excessive drainage or bleeding, skin necrosis, condition of drains.
  Drainage Volume: Note the volume and characteristics of drainage from Jackson-Pratt drain or other drains.
  Labs: Post-operative hematocrit value and other labs.
Assessment and Plan: Assess the patient's overall condition and status of wound. Comment on abnormal labs, and discuss treatment and discharge plans.

Postoperative Orders

1. **Transfer:** From recovery room to surgical ward when stable.
2. **Vital Signs:** q4h, I&O q4h x 24h.
3. **Activity:** Bed rest; ambulate in 6-8 hours if appropriate. Incentive spirometer q1h while awake.
4. **Diet:** NPO x 8h, then sips of water. Advance from clear liquids to regular diet as tolerated.
5. **IV Fluids:** IV D5 LR or D5 1/2 NS at 125 cc/h (KCL, 20 mEq/L if indicated), Foley to gravity.
6. **Medications:**
   Cefazolin (Ancef) 1 gm IVPB q8h x 3 doses; if indicated for prophylaxis in clean cases **OR**
   Cefotetan (Cefotan) 1 gm IV q12h x 2 doses for clean contaminated cases.
   Meperidine (Demerol) 50 mg IV/IM q3-4h prn pain
   Hydroxyzine (Vistaril) 25-50 mg IV/IM q3-4h prn nausea **OR**
   Prochlorperazine (Compazine) 10 mg IV/IM q4-6h prn nausea or suppository q 4h prn.
7. **Laboratory Evaluation:** CBC, SMA7, chest x-ray in AM if indicated.

Postoperative Surgical Management

I. **Postoperative day number 1**
   A. Assess the patient's level of pain, lungs, cardiac status, flatulence, and bowel movement. Examine for distension, tenderness, bowel sounds; wound drainage, bleeding from incision.
   B. Discontinue IV infusion when taking adequate PO fluids. Discontinue Foley catheter, and use in-and-out catheterization for urinary retention.
   C. Ambulate as tolerated; incentive spirometer, hematocrit and hemoglobin.
   D. Acetaminophen/codeine (Tylenol #3) 1-2 PO q4-6h prn pain.
   E. Colace 100 mg PO bid.
   F. Consider prophylaxis for deep vein thrombosis.

II. **Postoperative day number 2**
   A. If passing gas or if bowel movement, advance to regular diet unless bowel resection.
   B. Laxatives: Dulcolax suppository prn or Fleet enema prn or milk of magnesia, 30 cc PO prn constipation.

III. **Postoperative day number 3-7**
   A. Check pathology report.
   B. Remove staples and place steri-strips.
   C. Consider discharge home on appropriate medications; follow up in 1-2 weeks for removal of sutures.
   D. Write discharge orders (including prescriptions) in AM; arrange for home health care if indicated. Dictate discharge summary and send copy to surgeon and referring physician.

# Surgical Progress Note

Surgical progress notes are written in "SOAP" format.

Surgical Progress Note

Date/Time:
Post-operative Day Number:
Problem List: Antibiotic day number and hyperalimentation day number if applicable. List each surgical problem separately (eg, status-post appendectomy, hypokalemia).
Subjective: Describe how the patient feels in the patient's own words, and give observations about the patient. Indicate any new patient complaints, note the adequacy of pain relief, and passing of flatus or bowel movements. Type of food the patient is tolerating (eg, nothing, clear liquids, regular diet).
Objective:
    Vital Signs: Maximum temperature (T_{max}) over the past 24 hours. Current temperature, vital signs.
    Intake and Output: Volume of oral and intravenous fluids, volume of urine, stools, drains, and nasogastric output.
    Physical Exam:
        General appearance: Alert, ambulating.
        Heart: Regular rate and rhythm, no murmurs.
        Chest: Clear to auscultation.
        Abdomen: Bowel sounds present, soft, nontender.
        Wound Condition: Comment on the wound condition (eg, clean and dry, good granulation, serosanguinous drainage). Condition of dressings, purulent drainage, granulation tissue, erythema; condition of sutures, dehiscence. Amount and color of drainage
        Lab results: White count, hematocrit, and electrolytes, chest x-ray
Assessment and Plan: Evaluate each numbered problem separately. Note the patient's general condition (eg, improving), pertinent developments, and plans (eg, advance diet to regular, chest x-ray). For each numbered problem, discuss any additional orders and plans for discharge or transfer.

Procedure Note

A procedure note should be written in the chart when a procedure is performed. Procedure notes are brief operative notes.

Procedure Note

Date and time:
Procedure:
Indications:
Patient Consent: Document that the indications, risks and alternatives to the procedure were explained to the patient. Note that the patient was given the opportunity to ask questions and that the patient consented to the procedure in writing.
Lab tests: Electrolytes, INR, CBC
Anesthesia: Local with 2% lidocaine
Description of Procedure: Briefly describe the procedure, including sterile prep, anesthesia method, patient position, devices used, anatomic location of procedure, and outcome.
Complications and Estimated Blood Loss (EBL):
Disposition: Describe how the patient tolerated the procedure.
Specimens: Describe any specimens obtained and laboratory tests which were ordered.

Discharge Note

The discharge note should be written in the patient's chart prior to discharge.

Discharge Note

Date/time:
Diagnoses:
Treatment: Briefly describe treatment provided during hospitalization, including surgical procedures and antibiotic therapy.
Studies Performed: Electrocardiograms, CT scans, CXR.
Discharge Medications:
Follow-up Arrangements:

Discharge Summary

Patient's Name:
Chart Number:
Date of Admission:
Date of Discharge:
Admitting Diagnosis:
Discharge Diagnosis:
Name of Attending or Ward Service:
Surgical Procedures, Diagnostic Tests, Invasive Procedures:
Brief History and Pertinent Physical Examination and Laboratory Data: Describe the course of the patient's disease up to the time the patient came to the hospital, and describe the physical exam and pertinent laboratory data on admission.
Hospital Course: Briefly describe the course of the patient's illness while in the hospital, including evaluation, operation, outcome of the operation, and medications given while in the hospital.
Discharged Condition: Describe improvement or deterioration of the patient's condition.
Disposition: Describe the situation to which the patient will be discharged (home, nursing home) and the person who will provide care.
Discharged Medications: List medications and instructions and write prescriptions.
Discharged Instructions and Follow-up Care: Date of return for follow-up care at clinic; diet, exercise instructions.
Problem List: List all active and past problems.
Copies: Send copies to attending physician, clinic, consultants and referring physician.

Prescription Writing

- Patient's name:
- Date:
- Drug name, dosage form, dose, route, frequency (include concentration for oral liquids or mg strength for oral solids): Amoxicillin 125mg/5mL 5 mL PO tid
- Quantity to dispense: mL for oral liquids, # of oral solids
- Refills: If appropriate
- Signature

Clinical Care of the Surgical Patient

James G. Jakowitz, MD
Marianne Cinat, MD

Radiographic Evaluation of Common Interventions

I. **Central intravenous lines:**
   A. **Central venous catheters** should be located well above the right atrium, and not in a neck vein. Pneumothorax should be excluded by checking that the lung markings extend completely to the rib cages on both sides. An upright, expiratory x-ray may be helpful. Hemothorax will appear as opacification or a fluid meniscus on chest x-ray. Mediastinal widening may indicate great vessel injury.
   B. **Pulmonary artery catheters** should be located centrally and posteriorly and not more than 3-5 cm from midline within the mediastinum.

II. **Pulmonary tubes**
   A. **Endotracheal tubes:** Verify that the tube is located 3 cm below the vocal cords and 2-4 cm above the carina. The tip of tube should be at the level of aortic arch.
   B. **Tracheostomy:** Verify by chest x-ray that the tube is located half way between the stoma and the carina; the tube should be parallel to the long axis of the trachea. The tube should be approximately 2/3 of width of the trachea, and the cuff should not cause bulging of the trachea walls. Check for subcutaneous air in the neck tissue and for mediastinal widening secondary to air leakage.
   C. **Chest tubes:** A chest tube for pneumothorax drainage should be located anteriorly at the mid-clavicular line at the level of the third intercostal space or in the anterior axillary line directed toward the apex at the 4-5th intercostal space. Pleural effusions should be drained by locating the tube inferior-posteriorly at or about the level of the eighth intercostal space and directed posteriorly.
   D. **Mechanical ventilation:** A chest x-ray should be obtained to rule out pneumothorax, subcutaneous emphysema, pneumomediastinum or subpleural air cysts. Lung infiltrates may diminish or disappear because of increased aeration of the affected lung lobe.

III. **Gastrointestinal tubes**
   A. **Nasogastric tubes:** Verify that the tube is in the stomach and not coiled in the esophagus or trachea. The tip of the tube should not be near gastroesophageal junction. The standard size nasogastric tube is 14-16 French. Nasogastric tubes are used to decompress the stomach.
   B. **Feeding tubes** are smaller in size (8-12 Fr) than nasogastric tubes. They are flexible and are frequently used for enteral nutrition. They are passed nasally through the stomach and into the duodenum or jejunum. The tip is radiopaque, and it should be located in the distal stomach. The tube may extend through the pylorus into the duodenum.

Blood Component Therapy

I. **Crystalloids solutions:** Sodium is the principle component of crystalloid solutions, which is the most abundant solute in the extracellular fluid.
   A. **Hypotonic solutions** include 0.45% normal saline and 0.25% normal saline. Hypotonic solutions are used as maintenance fluids in adults (0.45% NS) and infants (0.25% NS).
   B. **Isotonic solutions** include normal saline (0.9% NaCl; 154 mEq Na and 154 mEq Cl) and lactated Ringers (130meq Na, 109 mEq Cl, 4 mEq K, 3 mEq Ca, lactate as a buffer). Isotonic solutions are used for acute resuscitation and volume replacement. Approximately 3 cc of crystalloid should be given to replace each 1 cc of blood loss.
   C. **Hypertonic saline** (7.5% NaCl; 1283 mEq Na, 1283 mEq Cl) is used to treat symptomatic hyponatremia. Replacement must be done slowly to prevent central pontine myelinolysis.

II. **Colloid solution therapy** is indicated for volume expansion.
   A. **Albumin (5% or 25%)** is useful for hypovolemia or to induce diuresis with furosemide in hypervolemic, hypoproteinemic patients. Salt poor albumin is used in cirrhosis.
   B. **Purified protein fraction (Plasmanate)** consists of 83% albumin and 17% globulin. It is indicated for volume expansion as an alternative to albumin.
   C. **Hetastarch (Hespan)** consists of synthetic colloid (6% hetastarch in saline). Hespan is useful for volume expansion and raising osmotic pressure. Maximum dose is 1500 cc per 24 hours. Hetastarch may prolong the partial thromboplastin time.

III. **Management of acute blood loss – red blood cell transfusions**
   A. Hemorrhage should be controlled, and crystalloids should be infused until packed red blood cells are available to replace losses. In trauma, bleeding may require surgical control. If crystalloids fail to produce hemodynamic stability after more than 2 liters have been administered, packed red blood cells should be given.
   B. If volume replacement and hemostasis stabilize the patient's hemodynamic status, formal type and cross match of blood should be completed. In exigent bleeding, O negative, low titer blood or type specific (ABO matched) Rh compatible blood should be administered.

IV. **Guidelines for blood transfusion in anemia.** Consider blood transfusion when hemoglobin is less than 8.0 gm/dL and hematocrit is less than 24%. If the patient has symptoms of anemia, such as chest pain, dyspnea, mental status changes, transfusion should be provided.

V. **Blood component products**
   A. **Packed red blood cells (PRBCs).** Each unit provides 400 cc of volume, and each unit should raise hemoglobin by 1 gm/dL and hematocrit by 3%.
   B. **Platelets** are indicated for bleeding due to thrombocytopenia or thrombopathy. Each unit should raise the platelet count by 5,000-10,000 cells/mul. Platelets are usually transfused 8-10 units at a time. Dilutional thrombocytopenia occurs after massive blood transfusions. Therefore, platelet transfusion should be considered after 8-10 units of blood replacement. ABO typing is not necessary before platelets are given.
   C. **Fresh frozen plasma (FFP)** is used for bleeding secondary to liver disease, dilutional coagulopathy (from multiple blood transfusions), or coagulation factor deficiencies. ABO typing is required before administration of FFP, but cross matching is not required. Improvement

of INR/PTT usually requires 2-3 units. One unit of FFP should be administered for every 4-6 units of PRBCs. FFP contains all clotting factors except factors V and VII.

D. **Cryoprecipitate** contains factor VIII, and fibrinogen. It is given 8-10 units at a time. Cryoprecipitate may be necessary for massive transfusions.

E. **Autologous blood.** The patient donates blood within 35 days of surgery; frozen blood can be stored for up to 2 years. Autologous blood is useful in elective orthopedic, cardiac, and peripheral vascular procedures.

Fluids and Electrolytes

I. **Maintenance fluid guidelines**
   A. Maintenance fluid requirements consist of 4 cc/kg for the first 10 kg of body weight, 2 cc/kg for the second 10 kg, and 1 cc/kg for each additional kg.
   B. A 70 mg patient has a maintenance fluid requirement of approximately 125 mL/hr. Maintenance fluids used are D5 1/2 NS with 20 mEq KCL/liter and D5 1/4 NS with 20 mEq KCl/liter in children.

II. **Pediatric patients**
   A. Use D5 1/4 NS with 20 mEq KCL/liter.
   B. 24 hour water requirement, kilogram method: For the first 10 kg body weight: 100 mL/kg/day PLUS for the second 10 kg body weight: 50 mL/kg/day PLUS for weight above 20 kg: 20 mL/kg/day. Divide by 24 hours to determine hourly rate.

III. **Specific replacement fluids of specific losses**
   A. **Gastric fluid (nasogastric tube, emesis).** D5 1/2 NS with 20 mEq/liter KCL; replace equal volume of lost fluid q6h.
   B. **Diarrhea.** D5LR with 15 mEq/liter KCL. Provide 1 liter replacement for each 1 kg or 2.2 lb of lost body weight; bicarbonate 45 mEq (1/2 amp) per liter may be added.
   C. **Bile.** D5LR with 25 mEq/liter (1/2 amp) of bicarbonate.
   D. **Pancreatic.** D5LR with 50 mEq/liter (1 amp) bicarbonate.

Evaluation of Postoperative Fever

I. **Clinical evaluation**
   A. **History.** Fever ≥100.4-101 F. Determine the number of days since operation.
   B. **Differential diagnosis.** Pneumonia, urinary tract infection, thrombophlebitis, wound infection, drug reaction. Atelectasis is the most common cause of fever less than 48 hrs after operation.
   C. Dysuria, abdominal pain, cough, sputum, headache, stiff neck, joint or back pain may be present.
   D. IV catheter infection (central or peripheral) is an important source of postoperative sepsis.
   E. **Fever pattern.** Check previous day for fever patterns; spiking fevers indicate abscesses. Continuous fevers or high fevers indicate vascular involvement, such as infected prosthetic grafts or septic phlebitis from central IV lines.
   F. Chills or rigors indicate bacteremia. These symptoms are usually not

associated with atelectasis or drug fevers.
  G. Fevers prior to the operation, alcohol use, allergies, and recent WBC count and differential counts should be assessed.

II. Physical Exam
  A. **General.** Temperature, fever curve, tachycardia, hypotension. Examine all vascular access sites carefully.
  B. **HEENT.** Pharyngeal erythema, neck rigidity.
  C. **Chest.** Rhonchi, crackles, dullness to percussion (pneumonia), murmurs (endocarditis).
  D. **Abdomen.** Masses, liver tenderness, Murphy's sign (right upper quadrant tenderness with inspiration, cholecystitis); ascites. Costovertebral angle or suprapubic tenderness. Examine wound for purulence, induration, or tenderness.
  E. **Extremities.** Infected decubitus ulcers or wounds; IV catheter tenderness (phlebitis); calf tenderness, joint tenderness (septic arthritis). Cellulitis, abscesses, perirectal abscess.
  F. **Genitourinary.** Prostate tenderness; rectal fluctuance. Cervical discharge, cervical motion tenderness; adnexal tenderness.

III. Laboratory evaluation.
CBC, blood C&S X 2, UA, urine C&S; blood, urine, sputum, wound cultures, chest x-ray.

IV. Differential diagnosis
  A. Wound infection, abscesses, intra-abdominal abscess, atelectasis, drug fever, pulmonary emboli, pancreatitis, alcohol withdrawal, deep vein thrombosis, tuberculosis, cystitis, pyelonephritis, osteomyelitis; IV catheter phlebitis, sinusitis, otitis media, upper respiratory infection, pelvic infection, cellulitis; hepatitis; infected decubitus ulcer, peritonitis, endocarditis, diverticulitis, cholangitis, carcinomas.
  B. **Medications associated with fever:** H2 blockers, penicillins, phenytoin, sulfonamides.

V. Antibiotics
should be initiated if there is any possibility of infection.

Sepsis

About 400,000 cases of sepsis, 200,000 cases of septic shock, and 100,000 deaths from both occur each year.

I. Pathophysiology
  A. Sepsis is defined as the systemic response to infection. In the absence of infection, it is called systemic inflammatory response syndrome and is characterized by at least two of the following: temperature greater than 38°C or less than 36°C; heart rate greater than 90 beats per minute; respiratory rate more than 20/minute or $PaCO_2$ less than 32 mm Hg; and an alteration in white blood cell count (>12,000/mm^3 or <4,000/mm^3).
  B. Septic shock is defined as sepsis-induced hypotension that persists despite fluid resuscitation and is associated with tissue hypoperfusion.
  C. The initial cardiovascular response to sepsis includes decreased systemic vascular resistance and depressed ventricular function. Low systemic vascular resistance occurs. If this initial cardiovascular response is uncompensated, generalized tissue hypoperfusion results. Aggressive fluid resuscitation may improve cardiac output and systemic blood pressure, resulting in the typical hemodynamic pattern of septic shock (ie, high cardiac index and low systemic vascular resistance).

D. Although gram-negative bacteremia is commonly found in patients with sepsis, gram-positive infection may affect 30-40% of patients. Fungal, viral and parasitic infections are usually encountered in immunocompromised patients.

Defining sepsis and related disorders

Term	Definition
Systemic inflammatory response syndrome (SIRS)	The systemic inflammatory response to a severe clinical insult manifested by ≥ 2 of the following conditions: Temperature >38°C or <36°C, heart rate >90 beats/min, respiratory rate >20 breaths/min or $PaCO_2$ <32 mm Hg, white blood cell count >12,000 cells/mm^3, <4000 cells/mm^3, or >10% band cells
Sepsis	The presence of SIRS caused by an infectious process; sepsis is considered severe if hypotension or systemic manifestations of hypoperfusion (lactic acidosis, oliguria, change in mental status) is present.
Septic shock	Sepsis-induced hypotension despite adequate fluid resuscitation, along with the presence of perfusion abnormalities that may induce lactic acidosis, oliguria, or an alteration in mental status.
Multiple organ dysfunction syndrome (MODS)	The presence of altered organ function in an acutely ill patient such that homeostasis cannot be maintained without intervention

E. Sources of bacteremia leading to sepsis include the urinary, respiratory and GI tracts, and skin and soft tissues (including catheter sites). The source of bacteremia is unknown in 30% of patients.

F. Escherichia coli is the most frequently encountered gram-negative organism, followed by Klebsiella pneumoniae, Enterobacter aerogenes or cloacae, Serratia marcescens, Pseudomonas aeruginosa, Proteus mirabilis, Providencia, and Bacteroides species. Up to 16% of sepsis cases are polymicrobic.

G. Gram-positive organisms, including methicillin-sensitive and methicillin-resistant Staphylococcus aureus and Staphylococcus epidermidis, are associated with catheter or line-related infections.

II. Diagnosis

A. A patient who is hypotensive and in shock should be evaluated to identify the site of infection, and monitor for end-organ dysfunction. History should be obtained and a physical examination performed.

B. **The early phases of septic shock** may produce evidence of volume depletion, such as dry mucous membranes, and cool, clammy skin. After resuscitation with fluids, however, the clinical picture resembles hyperdynamic shock, including tachycardia, bounding pulses with a widened pulse pressure, a hyperdynamic precordium on palpation, and warm extremities.

C. **Signs of infection** include fever, localized erythema or tenderness, consolidation on chest examination, abdominal tenderness, and meningismus. Signs of end-organ hypoperfusion include tachypnea, oliguria, cyanosis, mottling of the skin, digital ischemia, abdominal tenderness, and altered mental status.

- **D. Laboratory studies** should include arterial blood gases, lactic acid level, electrolytes, renal function, liver function tests, and chest radiograph. Cultures of blood, urine, and sputum should be obtained before antibiotics are administered. Cultures of pleural, peritoneal, and cerebrospinal fluid may be appropriate. If thrombocytopenia or bleeding is present, tests for disseminated intravascular coagulation should include fibrinogen, d-dimer assay, platelet count, peripheral smear for schistocytes, prothrombin time, and partial thromboplastin time.

Manifestations of Sepsis

Clinical features	Laboratory findings
Temperature instability	Respiratory alkaloses
Tachypnea	Hypoxemia
Hyperventilation	Increased serum lactate levels
Altered mental status	Leukocytosis and increased neutrophil concentration
Oliguria	Eosinopenia
Tachycardia	Thrombocytopenia
Peripheral vasodilation	Anemia
	Proteinuria
	Mildly elevated serum bilirubin levels

III. Treatment of septic shock

- **A.** Early management of septic shock is aimed at restoring mean arterial pressure to 65 to 75 mm Hg to improve organ perfusion. Continuous SVO₂ monitoring is recommended to insure optimal organ perfusion at the cellular level. Clinical clues to adequate tissue perfusion include skin temperature, mental status, and urine output. Urine output should be maintained at >20 to 30 mL/hr. 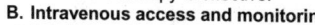 Lactic acid levels should decrease within 24 hours if therapy is effective.
- **B. Intravenous access and monitoring**
  1. Intravenous access is most rapidly obtained through peripheral sites with two 16- to 18-gauge catheters. More stable access can be achieved later with central intravenous access. Placement of a large-bore introducer catheter in the right internal jugular or left subclavian vein allows the most rapid rate of infusion.
  2. Arterial lines should be placed to allow for more reliable monitoring of blood pressure. Pulmonary artery catheters measure cardiac output, systemic vascular resistance, pulmonary artery wedge pressure, and mixed venous oxygen saturation. These data are useful in providing rapid assessment of response to various therapies.
- **C. Fluids**
  1. Aggressive volume resuscitation is essential in treatment of septic shock. Most patients require 4 to 8 L of crystalloid. Fluid should be administered as a bolus. The mean arterial pressure should be increased to 65 to 75 mm Hg and organ perfusion should be improved within 1 hour of the onset of hypotension.
  2. Repeated boluses of crystalloid (isotonic sodium chloride solution or lactated Ringer's injection), 500 to 1,000 mL, should be given intravenously over 5 to 10 minutes, until mean arterial pressure and tissue perfusion are adequate (about 4 to 8 L total over 24 hours for

the typical patient). Boluses of 250 mL are appropriate for patients who are elderly or who have heart disease or suspected pulmonary edema. Red blood cells should be reserved for patients with a hemoglobin value of less than 10 g/dL and either evidence of decreased oxygen delivery or significant risk from anemia (eg, coronary artery disease).

D. Vasoactive agents

1. Patients who do not respond to fluid therapy should receive vasoactive agents. The primary goal is to increase mean arterial pressure to 65 to 75 mm Hg.
2. **Dopamine (Intropin)** traditionally has been used as the initial therapy in hypotension, primarily because it is thought to increase systemic blood pressure. However, dopamine is a relatively weak vasoconstrictor in septic shock.

Hemodynamic effects of vasoactive agents

Agent	Dose	Effect		
		CO	MAP	SVR
Dopamine (Inotropin)	5-20 mcg/kg/min	2+	1+	3+
Norepinephrine (Levophed)	0.05-0.5 mcg/kg/min	-/0/+	2+	4+
Dobutamine (Dobutrex)	10 mcg/kg/min	2+	-/0/+	-/0
Epinephrine	0.05-2 mcg/kg/min	3+	2+	4+
Phenylephrine (Neo-Synephrine)	2-10 mcg/kg/min	0	2+	4+

3. **Norepinephrine (Levophed)** is superior to dopamine in the treatment of hypotension associated with septic shock. Norepinephrine is the agent of choice for treatment of hypotension related to septic shock.
4. **Dobutamine (Dobutrex)** should be reserved for patients with a persistently low cardiac index or underlying left ventricular dysfunction.

E. Antibiotics
should be administered within 2 hours of the recognition of sepsis. Use of vancomycin should be restricted to settings in which the causative agent is most likely resistant *Enterococcus*, methicillin-resistant *Staphylococcus aureus*, or high-level penicillin-resistant *Streptococcus pneumoniae*.

Recommended Antibiotics in Septic Shock

Suspected source	Recommended antibiotics
Pneumonia	Third or 4th-generation cephalosporin (cefepime, ceftazidime, cefotaxime, ceftizoxime) *plus* macrolide (antipseudomonal beta lactam *plus* aminoglycoside if hospital-acquired) ± anaerobic coverage with metronidazole or clindamycin.
Urinary tract	Ampicillin *plus* gentamicin (Garamycin) or third-generation cephalosporin (ceftazidime, cefotaxime, ceftizoxime) or a quinolone (ciprofloxacin, levofloxacin).
Skin or soft tissue	Nafcillin (add metronidazole [Flagyl] or clindamycin if anaerobic infection suspected)
Meningitis	Third-generation cephalosporin (ceftazidime, cefotaxime, ceftizoxime)
Intra-abdominal	Third-generation cephalosporin (ceftazidime, cefotaxime, ceftizoxime) *plus* metronidazole or clindamycin
Primary bacteremia	Ticarcillin/clavulanate (Timentin) *or* piperacillin/tazobactam (Zosyn)

Dosages of Antibiotics Used in Sepsis

Agent	Dosage
Cefepime (Maxipime)	2 gm IV q12h; if neutropenic, use 2 gm q8h
Ceftizoxime (Cefizox)	2 gm IV q8h
Ceftazidime (Fortaz)	2 g IV q8h
Cefotaxime (Claforan)	2 gm q4-6h
Cefuroxime (Kefurox, Zinacef)	1.5 g IV q8h
Cefoxitin (Mefoxin)	2 gm q6h
Cefotetan (Cefotan)	2 gm IV q12h
Piperacillin/tazobactam (Zosyn)	3.375-4.5 gm IV q6h
Ticarcillin/clavulanate (Timentin)	3.1 gm IV q4-6h (200-300 mg/kg/d)
Ampicillin	1-3.0 gm IV q6h
Ampicillin/sulbactam (Unasyn)	3.0 gm IV q6h
Nafcillin (Nafcil)	2 gm IV q4-6h

Sepsis

Agent	Dosage
Piperacillin, ticarcillin, mezlocillin	3 gm IV q4-6h
Meropenem (Merrem)	1 gm IV q8h
Imipenem/cilastatin (Primaxin)	1.0 gm IV q6h
Gentamicin or tobramycin	2 mg/kg IV loading dose, then 1.7 mg/kg IV q8h
Amikacin (Amikin)	7.5 mg/kg IV loading dose, then 5 mg/kg IV q8h
Vancomycin	1 gm IV q12h
Metronidazole (Flagyl)	500 mg IV q6-8h
Clindamycin (Cleocin)	600-900 mg IV q8h
Linezolid (Zyvox)	600 mg IV/PO q12h
Quinupristin/dalfopristin (Synercid)	7.5 mg/kg IV q8h

1. **Initial treatment of life-threatening sepsis** usually consists of a third or 4th-generation cephalosporin (cefepime, ceftazidime, cefotaxime, ceftizoxime) or piperacillin/tazobactam (Zosyn). An aminoglycoside (gentamicin, tobramycin, or amikacin) should also be included. Antipseudomonal coverage is important for hospital- or institutional-acquired infections. Appropriate choices include an antipseudomonal penicillin, cephalosporin, or an aminoglycoside.
2. **Methicillin-resistant staphylococci.** If line sepsis or an infected implanted device is a possibility, vancomycin should be added to the regimen to cover for methicillin-resistant Staph aureus and methicillin-resistant Staph epidermidis.
3. **Vancomycin-resistant enterococcus (VRE):** An increasing number of enterococcal strains are resistant to ampicillin and gentamicin. The incidence of vancomycin-resistant enterococcus (VRE) is rapidly increasing.
   a. **Linezolid (Zyvox)** is an oral or parenteral agent active against vancomycin-resistant enterococci, including E. faecium and E. faecalis. Linezolid is also active against methicillin-resistant staphylococcus aureus.
   b. **Quinupristin/dalfopristin (Synercid)** is a parenteral agent active against strains of vancomycin-resistant enterococcus faecium, but not enterococcus faecalis. Most strains of VRE are enterococcus faecium.
F. **Other therapies**
   1. **Hydrocortisone** (100 mg every 8 hours) in patients with refractory shock significantly improves hemodynamics and survival rates. Corticosteroids may be beneficial in patients with refractory shock caused by an Addison's crisis.
   2. **Activated protein C (drotrecogin alfa [Xigris])** has antithrombotic,

profibrinolytic, and anti-inflammatory properties. Activated protein C reduces the risk of death by 20%. Activated protein C is approved for treatment of patients with severe sepsis who are at high risk of death. Drotrecogin alfa is administered as 24 mcg/kg/hr for 96 hours. There is a small risk of bleeding. Contraindications are thrombocytopenia, coagulopathy, recent surgery or recent hemorrhage.

References: See page 113.

Nutrition in the Surgical Patient

I. **Nutritional requirements** are based on the patient's nutritional needs, stress and severity of illness. Requirements are divided into non-protein calories per kilogram (npc/kg) and grams of protein per kilogram (gm protein/kg) per 24-hour period.

Nutritional Requirements		
Patient	Non-protein calories/kg	Protein
Well-nourished, unstressed	20-25 npc/kg/day	1 gm/kg
Minimal stress (post-op)	25-30 npc/kg/day	1-1.2 gm/kg
Moderate stress (multiple trauma, infection)	30-35 npc/kg/day	1.2-1.5 gm/kg
Severe stress (severe sepsis, critical illness)	35-40 npc/kg/day	1.5-2.0 gm/kg
Extreme stress (burns> 40% body surface area)	40-45 npc/kg/day	2.0-2.5 gm/kg

A. **Sources of non-protein calories**
   1. **Carbohydrate solutions** contain dextrose, which contains 3.4 kcal/gm
   2. **Lipid solutions** contain 9.1 kcal/gm
B. **Protein calories.** Amino acid solutions contain protein in a concentration of 4 kcal/gm

II. **Enteral nutrition**
   A. Enteral nutrition is more physiologic and technically easier to administer than parenteral nutrition. Enteral nutrition can be administered via nasogastric, nasoduodenal or nasojejunal tubes, or gastrostomy or jejunostomy tubes.
   B. **Continuous enteral infusion**
      1. Initial enteral solution infusion starts at 30 m/hr. Increase rate by 30 mL

at 4-hour intervals as tolerated until the final rate is achieved. Residual volume should be measured every 4 hours; hold feedings for 1 hour if the residual is greater than 2 times the infusion rate.
2. **Gastric/duodenal feedings:** Start with full strength formula and increase the rate until the goal is achieved.
3. **Jejunal feedings:** Start with 1/4 strength formula. Increase the rate until the goal is achieved. Once at goal rate, change to 1/2 strength formula for 4-8 hours, then ¾ strength formula for 4-8 hours, then full strength formula for 4-8 hours. This method allows the mucosa of the distal small bowel to adjust to the increased osmolarity of enteral formulas.

C. **Bolus feedings:** Give 50-100 cc enteral nutrition every 3 hours initially. Increase by 50 cc each feeding until the goal of 250-300 cc q 3-4 hours is achieved. Flush tube with 100 cc of water after each bolus.

D. **Promotility agents** are given to improve gastric emptying
1. Metoclopramide (Reglan) 5-10 mg PO/IV q6h **OR**
2. Erythromycin 125 mg IV or via nasogastric tube q8h.

E. **Antidiarrheal Agents**
1. Loperamide (Imodium) 2-4 mg q6h.
2. Diphenoxylate/atropine (Lomotil) 2.5-5.0 mg q4-6h.

Total Parental Nutrition

I. **Indications for total parenteral nutritions:** Prolonged post-operative ileus, inability to take oral feedings for more than 5 days, severe malnutrition, intestinal fistula, pancreatitis. Total parenteral nutrition should be given via a central catheter because of high osmolality.

II. **Standard solutions and components**
   A. **Dextrose solutions.** Various concentrations are available. One gram of dextrose yields 3.4 kcal.

Dextrose Solutions		
Solution	Concentration	Calories
10%	100 gm/liter	340 kcal/liter
20%	200 gm/liter	680 kcal/liter
50%	500 gm/liter	1700 kcal/liter
70%	700 gm/liter	2380 kcal/liter

   B. **Lipid solutions** consist of lipid emulsions of long-chain triglycerides. These are usually given in 500 cc volumes at 32 cc/hour for 16 hours.

Total Parental Nutrition 25

Lipid Solutions

Solution	Concentration	Calories
10%	50 gm/500 cc	500 kcal
20%	100 gm-500 cc	1000 kcal

C. Amino acid solutions supply protein. Various types of solutions at various concentrations are available.

Amino Acid Solutions

Solution	Concentration	Indications
Aminosyn 7%	70 gm/liter	Standard
Aminosyn-HBC* 7%	70 gm/liter	Hypercatabolism
Aminosyn-RF 5.2%	52 gm/liter	Renal Failure
HepatAmine 8%	80 gm/liter	Liver Failure
FreAmine 10%	100 gm/liter	Fluid Overload (highly concentrated)

*__High-branched chain aminoacid formulas__ may prevent muscle breakdown and may prevent hepatic encephalopathy.

D. Electrolyte requirements should be adjusted daily based on patient labs.

Electrolyte Requirements

Usual concentration	Range
Sodium 60 (meg/L)	0-150 meq/L
Potassium 20 (meg/L)	0-80 meq/L
Acetate* 50 (meg/L)	50-150 meq/L
Chloride 50 (meg/L)	0-150 meq/L
Phosphate 15 (meg/L)	0-30 meq/L
Calcium** 4.5 (meg/L)	0-20 meq/L
Magnesium 5.0 (meg/L)	5-15 meq/L

26 Total Parental Nutrition

> * Acetate is used in addition to chloride to help prevent hyperchloremic acidosis. One-third to one half of sodium and potassium should be supplied in the form of acetate rather than chloride.
> ** Calcium should be given as calcium gluconate or calcium chloride. One gram of calcium supplies 4.5 meq of calcium.

1. Other additives
   a. **Multivitamins** 1 amp daily
   b. **Vitamin K** 10 mg each week
   c. **Trace elements** chromium, copper, manganese, zinc, selenium

E. Ordering Total Parenteral Nutrition
   1. **Step One.** Determine the daily non-protein calories (dextrose and lipid) and grams or protein (amino acid) that the patient needs.

   Non-protein calory requirement/kg/day = wt in kg x npc requirement/kg/d

   Protein requirement = wt in kg x protein requirement/kg/d

   2. **Step Two.** Non-protein calories consist of lipids and carbohydrate (dextrose) solutions. The amount of each component should be determined. 500cc of 10% Intralipid solution will supply approximately 500 npc kcal. The patient will require the remaining non-protein calories from the dextrose solution. If using D50, the volume of D50 = npc x 1000 cc/1700 kcal.

   3. **Step Three.** Protein calories are supplied by amino acid solutions.

   Vol of 7% Aminosyn = gm protein required/d x 100 cc/7 gm

   4. **Step Four.** Combine the above volumes to determine total volume and rate. The dextrose and amino acid solutions are mixed together and given over 24 hours. The lipid solution is infused separately over 24 hours.

F. Methods of delivery
   1. **Continuous infusion of the solutions** over 24 hours is the most common method of administration. The TPN solution should be initiated slowly at 40 cc/hr for the first 24 hours. The rate can then be gradually increased by 30 cc/hr every four hours until the goal rate is reached.
   2. **Cyclic total parenteral nutrition 12-hour night schedule.** Taper continuous infusion in the morning by reducing the rate to half of the original rate for one hour. Further reduce the rate by half for an additional hour, then discontinue. Restart TPN in the afternoon. Taper at the beginning and end of cycle.

G. Laboratory examinations
   1. **Baseline Labs:** CBC, electrolytes, liver function tests, prealbumin, transferrin, triglyceride level, chest x-ray for line placement
   2. **Daily Labs:** Electrolytes, calcium, phosphorous until stable; glucometer checks with insulin sliding scale every 4–6 hours
   3. **Weekly Labs:** CBC, electrolytes, calcium, phosphorous, liver function tests, triglyceride level (4-6 hours after completion of lipid infusion; should be maintained <200 mg/dl)

4. **Nutritional Assessment** to determine adequacy of nutritional supplementation:
   a. Prealbumin or transferrin weekly
   b. 24-hour urine for urine urea nitrogen (to calculate nitrogen balance
III. **Peripheral parenteral nutrition (PPN)** can be delivered via peripheral veins.
   A. The goal of PPN is to provide enough non-protein calories to prevent catabolism and the breakdown of visceral proteins. Peripheral parenteral nutrition is not meant to create a positive nitrogen balance or anabolic state, and it should be used for short-term support only.
   B. PPN usually consists of a 3% amino acid solution mixed with dextrose 20% or glycerol. Intralipids (10% or 20%) can also be given peripherally to supply extra calories.

Central Venous Catheterization

I. **Indications for central venous catheter cannulation:** Monitoring of central venous pressures in shock or heart failure; management of fluid status; administration of total parenteral nutrition; prolonged antimicrobial therapy or chemotherapy.

II. **Location of catheterization site**
   A. The internal jugular approach should not be used in patients with a carotid bruit, carotid stenosis, or an aneurysm.
   B. The subclavian approach should be avoided in patients with emphysema or bullae.
   C. The external jugular or internal jugular approach by direct cut-down may be preferable in patients with coagulopathy or thrombocytopenia.
   D. If a chest tube already in place, the catheter should be placed on the same side as the chest tube.

III. **Technique of insertion into the external jugular vein**
   A. The external jugular vein courses from the angle of the mandible to behind the middle of clavicle, where it joins with the subclavian vein. Place patient in Trendelenburg's position, and apply digital pressure to the external jugular vein above clavicle to distend the vein. Cleanse the skin with Betadine iodine solution using sterile technique. Inject 1% lidocaine to produce a skin weal.
   B. With an 18-gauge, thin-wall needle, advance the needle into the vein. Then pass a J-guidewire through the needle; the wire should advance without resistance. Remove the needle, maintaining control over the guidewire at all times. Nick the skin with a No. 11 scalpel blade.
   C. With guidewire in place, pass the central catheter over the wire, and remove the guidewire after the catheter is in place. Cover the catheter hub with a finger to prevent air embolization.
   D. Attach a syringe to the catheter hub, and ensure that there is free backflow of dark venous blood. Attach the catheter to an intravenous infusion at a keep open rate. Secure the catheter in place with 2-0 silk suture and tape.
   E. Obtain a chest x-ray to confirm position and rule out pneumothorax. The catheter should be removed and changed within 3-4 days.

IV. **Internal jugular vein cannulation.** The internal jugular vein is positioned behind the sternocleidomastoid muscle, lateral to the carotid artery. The catheter should be placed at a location at the upper confluence of the two

bellies of sternocleidomastoid at the level of cricoid cartilage.
- A. Place the patient in Trendelenburg's position, and turn the patient's head to the contralateral side. Choose a location on the right or left. If lung function is symmetrical and no chest tubes are in place, the right side is preferred because of the direct path to the superior vena cava. Prepare the skin with Betadine solution using sterile technique and drape the area. Infiltrate the skin and deeper tissues with 1% lidocaine.
- B. Palpate the carotid artery. Using a 22-gauge scout needle and syringe, direct the needle toward the ipsilateral nipple at a 30 degree angle to the neck. While aspirating, advance the needle until the vein is located and blood back flows into the syringe.
- C. Remove the scout needle and advance an 18-gauge, thin wall, catheter-over-needle (with an attached syringe) along the same path as the scout needle. When back flow of blood is noted into the syringe, advance the catheter into the vein. Remove the needle and confirm back flow of blood through the catheter and into the syringe. Remove the syringe and cover the catheter hub with a finger to prevent air embolization.
- D. With the catheter in position, advance a guidewire through the catheter. The guidewire should advance easily without resistance.
- E. With the guidewire in position, remove the catheter and use a No. 11 scalpel blade to nick the skin. Place the central vein catheter over the wire, holding the wire secure at all times. Pass the catheter into the vein, and suture the catheter to the skin with O silk suture. Tape the catheter in place, and connect it to an IV infusion at a keep open rate.
- F. Obtain a chest x-ray to rule out pneumothorax and confirm position.

V. Subclavian vein cannulation
- A. The subclavian vein is located in the angle formed by the medial 1/3 of clavicle and the first rib.
- B. Position the patient supine with a rolled towel located longitudinally between the patient's scapulae, and turn the patient's head towards the contralateral side. Prepare the area with Betadine iodine solution, and, using sterile technique, drape the area and infiltrate 1% lidocaine into the skin and tissues.
- C. Use a 16-gauge needle, with syringe attached, to puncture the mid-point of the clavicle, advancing until the clavicle bone and needle come in contact.
- D. Then slowly probe down until the needle slips under the clavicle. Advance the needle slowly towards the vein until the needle enters the vein, and a back flow of venous blood enters the syringe. Remove the syringe, and cover the catheter hub with a finger to prevent air embolization.
- E. With the 16-gauge catheter in position, advance a 0.89 mm x 45 cm guidewire through the catheter. The guidewire should advance easily without resistance. With the guidewire in position, remove the catheter, and use a No. 11 scalpel blade to nick the skin. Pass the dilator over the wire.
- F. Place the central line catheter over the wire, holding the wire secure at all times. Pass the catheter into the vein, and suture the catheter to the skin with 2-0 silk suture, tape the catheter in place and connect to IV infusion. Obtain a chest x-ray to confirm the position of the catheter tip and rule out pneumothorax.

Pulmonary Artery Catheterization

1. Cannulate a vein using the technique above, such as the subclavian vein or internal jugular. Advance a guidewire through the cannula, and remove the cannula. Nick the skin with a number 11 scalpel blade adjacent to the guidewire, and pass a number 8 French introducer over the wire and into the vein. Connect the introducer to an IV fluid infusion at a keep open rate, and suture introducer to the skin with 2-0 silk.
3. Pass the proximal end of the pulmonary artery catheter (Swan Ganz) to an assistant for connection to a continuous flush transducer system.
4. Flush the distal and proximal ports with heparin solution, removing all bubbles, and check balloon integrity by inflating 2 cc of air. Check pressure transducer response by moving the distal tip quickly.
5. Pass the catheter through the introducer into the vein 10-20 cm, then inflate the balloon, and advance the catheter until the balloon is in or near the right atrium.
6. The correct distance to the entrance of the right atrium is determined from the site of insertion:
   Right antecubital fossa: 35-40 cm.
   Left antecubital fossa: 45-50 cm.
   Right internal jugular vein: 10-15 cm.
   Subclavian vein: 10 cm.
   Femoral vein: 35-45 cm.
7. Run a continuous monitoring strip to record pressures as the PA catheter is advanced. Advance the balloon, inflated with 0.8-1.0 cc of air, while monitoring pressures and wave forms. Advance the catheter through the right ventricle into the main pulmonary artery until the catheter enters a distal branch of the pulmonary artery and is stopped by impaction (as evidenced by a pulmonary wedge pressure wave form).
8. Do not advance catheter with balloon deflated, and do not withdraw the catheter with the balloon inflated. After placement, obtain a chest x-ray to verify that the tip of catheter is no farther than 3-5 cm from the midline, and no pneumothorax is present.

Normal Pulmonary Artery Catheter Values

Right atrial pressure	1-7 mmHg
RVP Systolic	15-25 mmHg
RVP Diastolic	8-15 mmHg
Pulmonary artery pressure	
PAP Systolic	15-25 mmHg
PAP Diastolic	8-15 mmHg
PAP Mean	10-20 mmHg
PCWP	6-12 mmHg
Cardiac Output	3.5-5.5 L/min
Cardiac Index	2.0-3.2 L/min/m^2
Systemic Vascular Resistance	800-1200 dyne/sec/cm^2

Venous Cutdown

Procedures
1. Obtain a venous cutdown tray, or a minor procedure tray and instrument tray with a silk suture (3-0, 4-0) and a catheter. This procedure will require sterile gloves, sterile towels/drapes, 4x4 gauze sponges, povidone-iodine solution, 5 cc syringe, 25 gauge needle, 1% lidocaine with epinephrine, adhesive tape, scissors, needle holder, hemostat, scalpel and blade, 3-O or 4-O silk suture.
2. Apply a tourniquet proximal to the site, and identify the vein. Remove the tourniquet and prep the skin with povidone-iodine solution and drape the area. Infiltrate the skin with 1% lidocaine, then incise the skin transversely.
3. Spread the incision long-wise in the direction of the vein with a hemostat and dissect adherent tissue from the vein. Lift the vein and pass two chromic or silk ties (3-0 or 4-0) behind the vein.
4. Tie off the distal suture, using the upper tie for traction. Make a transverse nick in the vein. If necessary, use a catheter introducer to hold the lumen of the vein open.
5. Make a small stab incision in the skin distal to the main skin incision, and insert a plastic catheter or IV cannula through the incision, then insert it into vein. Tie the proximal suture, and attach an infusion of IV fluid. Release the tourniquet. Suture the skin with silk or nylon, and apply a dressing.

Arterial Line Placement

Procedure
1. Obtain a 20 gauge, 1 1/2-2 inch, catheter-over-needle assembly (Angiocath), arterial line setup (transducer, tubing, pressure bag containing heparinized saline), armboard, sterile dressing, 1% lidocaine, 3 cc syringe, 25 gauge needle, and 3-0 silk.
2. The radial artery should be used. Use the Allen test to verify patency of the radial artery and adequacy of ulnar artery collaterals. Place the extremity on an armboard with a gauze roll behind the wrist to maintain hyperextension.
3. Prep with povidone-iodine and drape the wrist area. Infiltrate 1% lidocaine using a 25 gauge needle. Choose a site where the artery is most superficial and as distal as possible on the wrist.
4. Palpate the artery with the left hand, and use other hand to advance a 20 gauge catheter-over-needle into the artery at a 30 degree angle to the skin. When a flash of blood is seen, hold the needle in place and advance the catheter into the artery; occlude the artery with manual pressure while pressure tubing is connected.
5. If a needle and guide-wire kit is used, advance the guidewire into the artery, and pass the catheter over the guide-wire.
6. Suture the catheter in place with 3-0 silk, and apply a dressing.

Cricothyrotomy

I. Needle cricothyrotomy
A. Obtain a 12-14 gauge, catheter-over-needle (Angiocath or Jelco), 6-12 mL syringe, 3 mm pediatric endotracheal tube adapter, oxygen tubing, and a high flow oxygen source.
B. Locate the cricothyroid membrane (the notch between the thyroid cartilage and cricoid cartilage). Cleanse the neck area with povidone-iodine solution, and inject 2% lidocaine with epinephrine if the patient is conscious.
C. With a 12 or 14 gauge, catheter-over-needle assembly on the syringe, advance needle through the cricothyroid membrane at a 45 degree angle directed inferiorly. Apply back pressure on the syringe until air is aspirated.
D. Advance the catheter and remove the needle, then attach the hub to a 3 mm endotracheal tube adapter connected to oxygen tubing.
E. Administer oxygen at 15 liters per minute for 1-2 seconds on, then 4 seconds off. Air flow is controlled with a Y-connector or a hole in the side of the tubing.
F. The needle cricothyrotomy should be replaced with oral endotracheal intubation as soon as possible. A needle cricothyrotomy should not be used for more than 45 minutes, since exhalation of CO_2 is inadequate.

II. Surgical cricothyrotomy
A. Obtain a #5-#7 tracheostomy tube; tracheostomy tube adapter to connect to bag-mask ventilator; povidone-iodine solution, sterile gauze pads, scalpel handle, and hemostat.
B. Clean the neck area with povidone-iodine. Locate the thyroid and cricoid cartilages; the cricothyroid membrane extends between these two cartilages.
C. Infiltrate the overlying skin with 2% lidocaine with epinephrine if the patient is conscious. Stabilize the thyroid cartilage with the left hand, and make a vertical incision through the skin and subcutaneous tissues overlying the cricothyroid membrane, avoiding the large vessels that are located laterally.
D. Make a stab incision inferiorly in the cricothyroid membrane with the point of the blade. Insert the knife handle, and rotate the handle 90 degrees to open the incision; or use a hemostat to dilate the opening. Gently insert the endotracheal tube and secure with tape. A tracheostomy tube or an endotracheal tube may be used.
E. The surgical cricothyrotomy should be replaced with a formal tracheostomy within 24 hours.

References: See page 113.

Trauma

Michael E. Lekawa, MD

Management of the Trauma Patient

I. **Primary Survey of the Trauma Patient:** The primary survey should identify immediate life threatening injuries.
   - A = Assess airway maintenance with cervical spine protection.
   - B = Assess breathing and administer assisted ventilation if required; rule out tension pneumothorax. *breath sounds equal?*
   - C = Assess circulation and control hemorrhage. *BP, pulses*
   - D = Assess disability and neurologic status (determine the level of consciousness with Glasgow Coma Scale).
   - E = Exposure: Completely undress the patient and prevent hypothermia.

II. **Resuscitation phase:** The primary survey and resuscitation of the patient should be done simultaneously.
   - A. Assess airway and alleviate obstruction. Establish a definitive airway for patients with a GCS of less than 8 or hemodynamic instability. Protect the cervical spine until fractures have been excluded.
   - B. Give oxygen and manage tension pneumothorax with needle or tube thoracostomy.
   - C. Control hemorrhage by direct pressure or by surgical ligation. At least 2 large bore IVs should be places, and infuse 2-3 liters of warm Ringer's lactate solution (LR) as needed. Administer type specific or O-negative blood if the response to LR is inadequate. Send blood for type and cross and hemoglobin.
   - D. If the patient has a decreased level of consciousness, treat hypoxemia and shock, and evaluate for intracranial space-occupying lesion.
   - E. Give warm fluids, keep the room warm, and cover the patient with warm blankets. Small doses of short acting narcotics (Fentanyl) or benzodiazepines may be given as needed.

III. **Ongoing assessment and treatment**
   - A. Change to cross matched blood when available.
   - B. Monitor for coagulopathy. The PT/PTT and fibrinogen level should be monitored, and fresh frozen plasma, cryoprecipitate or platelets should be administered as indicated.
   - C. A nasogastric tube should be placed for decompression of the stomach (caution if facial fracture or unstable cervical spine).
   - D. **Shock**
     1. A Foley catheter should be placed to evaluate urine output. Adequate resuscitation is suggested by improvement in physiologic parameters such as heart rate, systolic pressure, ventilatory rate, distal perfusion and capillary refill, pulse oximetry, arterial blood gas, and urine output.
     2. Reassess ABCs prior to beginning secondary survey.

IV. **Secondary survey**
   - A. Obtain an abbreviated history, including allergies, medications, past illness, last meal, event/mechanism (AMPLE history).
   - B. Evaluate the completely undressed patient, front and back, and from head to toe. Evaluate each system (head and neck, chest, abdomen, perineum, musculoskeletal, vascular and neurologic).

C. Obtain x-rays of the chest, cervical spine, and pelvis. Perform peritoneal lavage, and/or CT-scan as needed. Unstable patients should not be sent to the radiology department.
D. **Laboratory studies:** Send type and cross for six units or more of packed red blood cells; complete blood count, platelet count, creatinine, glucose, ethanol level, pregnancy test, arterial blood gasses, UA, and urine toxicology screens.

V. Treatment of shock

A. **Maintain airway, breathing, and circulation (ABCs).** Rapid exsanguinating injuries take precedence over other injuries, including head injuries.
B. **Initial stabilization:** Control external bleeding with direct external pressure. Place two 14 or 16 gauge intravenous lines and type and cross for packed red blood cells. If there is insufficient time to cross match, give type O-negative blood. Type specific blood should be given if time permits.
C. For hypotensive patients, give an initial fluid challenge of 2 liters of LR over 5-10 min or 20 ml/kg in children over 5-10 min. Assess response to initial fluid challenge by checking blood pressure and heart rate. Patients who respond with only a transient increase in blood pressure should be rechallenged with LR or blood transfusion. Blood loss may be continuing in these patients.
D. Patients who do not respond to initial fluid challenge may have had either extensive blood loss or continuing bleeding, which must be identified (chest, abdomen, extremities, pelvis). Surgical intervention should be initiated. Other causes of hypotension include tension pneumothorax and cardiac tamponade.

VI. Empiric management of coagulopathy.
Consider empiric administration of 1 unit FFP for every 4 units of packed red blood cells, and consider 10 units platelets (or 1 unit of single donor platelets) per 6 units PRBC.

Penetrating Abdominal Trauma

I. Gun shot wounds

A. All abdominal gun shot wounds require exploratory laparotomy. Tangential wounds that do not penetrate the peritoneal cavity may be assessed by peritoneal lavage or laparoscopy if the wound is located on the anterior abdominal wall.

II. Stab wounds and other penetrating abdominal trauma

A. Exploratory laparotomy is required if an acute abdomen is present or if signs of visceral injury, shock, hypertension, upper or lower GI bleeding, evisceration or pneumoperitoneum is present.
B. If the patient is stable and the abdominal fascia has been penetrated or if disruption cannot be ruled out by local exploration, diagnostic peritoneal lavage (DPL) or 24 hours of serial exams should be completed.
C. Consider tetanus prophylaxis as indicated.

Blunt Abdominal Trauma

I. Physical findings of peritonitis or pneumoperitoneum on x-ray require exploratory laparotomy.
II. **If the patient has a non-acute abdomen**
   A. If the patient is stable with a clinically evaluable abdomen who does not undergo exploratory laparotomy, serial abdominal exams should be performed. If significant tenderness or peritoneal signs are noted, the patient should be evaluated by diagnostic peritoneal lavage, CT, or laparotomy.
   B. If the clinical evaluation is inadequate, perform diagnostic peritoneal lavage or CT-scan to rule out intra-abdominal injury.
   C. If the patient is not stable (systolic blood pressure <100 mmHg, HR >100, decreasing hemoglobin) and abdominal injury is possible, diagnostic peritoneal lavage should be done rather than CT-scan. If lavage is positive, laparotomy is required.
   D. If a CT-scan shows isolated splenic or liver injury, and the patient remains stable, the patient may be observed in the ICU. Other injuries should be assessed with laparotomy. CT-scan is less sensitive for intestinal or diaphragmatic injury.
   E. If there is a significant head injury, intoxication, or distracting injury (eg, multiple rib fractures, pelvic fracture, extremity fracture), the abdominal exam is unreliable. These patients must be evaluated by diagnostic peritoneal lavage or CT-scan.
   F. If the patient is to undergo a prolonged orthopedic or neurosurgical procedure, the abdomen should be evaluated with diagnostic peritoneal lavage or CT-scan before the procedure. A diagnostic peritoneal lavage can be done in the operating room.
III. **Diagnostic peritoneal lavage**
   A. Insert a nasogastric tube and Foley catheter to decompress the stomach and the bladder. Restrain or sedate the patient if necessary. Prep and drape the periumbilical region with Betadine solution and sterile towels. A site should be selected above or below umbilicus. If the patient has a pelvic fracture or if pregnant, the site should be located above the umbilicus.
   B. Infiltrate the skin and subcutaneous tissue with 1% lidocaine with epinephrine. Incise the skin with a 1.5 cm vertical incision through the subcutaneous tissue down to fascia. Use a No. 11 scalpel blade to make a 2-3 mm stab incision into the fascia. Apply traction to both sides of fascial incision with towel clips. An assistant should apply strong upward traction on clips. Dissect bluntly with a small hemostat to the peritoneum, then grasp and incise the peritoneum, and introduce a lavage catheter into the pelvis.
   C. Aspirate with a 12 cc syringe. If 10 cc of blood is returned, the lavage should be considered "grossly positive" which mandates an immediate laparotomy. If the aspirate is negative, instill 1 liter of LR or saline from a pressure bag. Periodically agitate the abdomen. When only a small amount of fluid remains in the bag, drop bag to the floor, and drain the fluid by siphon action.
   D. During the procedure, keep a sponge packed in the wound and hold the catheter in place. After at least 400 cc of fluid have been removed, clamp the tubing and withdraw the catheter. Close the fascial defect with heavy absorbable suture, and staple the skin.

E. Previous abdominal surgery, morbid obesity and advanced cirrhosis are relative contraindication to diagnostic peritoneal lavage. If diagnostic peritoneal lavage is indicated, it should be done by open, rather than the closed, Seldinger technique.

IV. Criteria for a positive peritoneal lavage
A. Gross blood; red blood cell count <100,000 cells/mm^3 (or 5-10,000 cells/mm^3) white blood cell count >500 cells/mm^3. Presence of food particles, bile, feces, or bacteria on Gram stain. Exit of lavage fluid via a chest tube or bladder catheter.

B. Amylase >20 IU/L; alkaline phosphates >3 IU.

Head Trauma

I. Initial management of head trauma
A. Support airway, breathing, and circulation (ABCs). A cervical spine injury should be considered to be present in any patient with multisystem trauma.

B. Intravenous resuscitation solutions should consist of isotonic Ringer's lactate (LR) or normal saline (NS). Fluids should be infused until the patient is euvolemic.

C. Make an initial assessment of the patient during the primary survey (alert, voice, pain, unresponsive).

D. Perform a mini-neurologic examination and repeat frequently (GCS, motor/lateralizing signs).

E. A history, including the mechanism of injury, past medical history, drug intake, should be completed.

Glasgow Coma Scale Assessment of Level of Consciousness	
Eye Opening	**Points**
Spontaneous	4
To speech	3
To pain	2
None	1
Verbal Response	
Oriented	5
Confused	4
Inappropriate words	3
Incomprehensible sounds	2
None	1

36 Head Trauma

Best Motor Response	
Obeys	6
Localities	5
Withdraws	4
Flexion	3
Extension	2
None	1

- **F.** Examine the skull depressed skull fractures, Battle's sign (blood in the ear canal or ecchymosis over mastoid process), Raccoon's eyes (periorbital ecchymosis), or rhinorrhea. If any of these signs are present, the patient requires admission and a neurosurgical consult. Nasogastric and nasotracheal intubation are contraindicated in patients with significant facial trauma because a cribriform plate fracture may be present.

II. Secondary management of head trauma
- **A.** All patients with significant head trauma should be admitted for at least 24 hours of serial neurological exams unless Glasgow coma scale is 15 and there is only brief amnesia of events, without loss of consciousness. Such patients may be discharged with instructions if reliable observation is ensured.
- **B.** If the Glasgow coma scale is 14 or less, or if loss of consciousness was for more than a few seconds, a head CT-scan should be obtained.
- **C.** If the mechanism of injury was significantly violent (rollover of vehicle) or if massive upper torso trauma, or if any lateralizing neurologic deficits, a head CT-scan should be obtained.
- **D.** If the Glasgow coma scale is less than 8 or if unequal pupils, lateralizing deficits, or open head injury, there is a high probability of a subdural, epidural, or intracerebral bleed or diffuse axonal injury. This patient requires ICU admission after obtaining a CT-scan of the head and a neurosurgical consultation.

III. Ongoing management of head trauma
- **A.** Continually reassess ABCs, ECG, systolic blood pressure, heart rate, and pulse oximeter. Serial hemoglobin or hematocrit should be obtained.
- **B.** Isolated head injuries rarely cause hypotension. If hypotension is present, the cause should be vigorously sought. Secondary causes of brain injury, such as hypoxia and hypotension, should be managed immediately.
- **C.** Stress ulcer prophylaxis with H_2-blockers (ranitidine, cimetidine) or sucralfate should be administered.
- **D.** Sequential compression stockings should be applied if the Glasgow coma scale is less than 13, or if spinal cord injury or pharmacologic paralysis is present.
- **E.** Mannitol 1 gm/kg is used to treat elevated intracranial pressure, especially in normotensive patients with pupillary abnormalities, or lateralizing signs. Steroids are not indicated in acute head injuries. Hyperventilation may be used for short periods in select patients.
- **F.** Open head wounds should be cleaned and repaired.
- **G.** Tetanus prophylaxis should be given with 0.5 cc tetanus toxoid IM, with

or without tetanus Ig 250 IU, IM, as indicated.
- H. Patients with an abnormal head CT-scan, neurologic deficit or a sustained Glasgow coma scale less than 14 require early neurosurgery consultation.

Thoracic Trauma

I. Management of traumatic pneumothorax
- A. Give high-flow oxygen and immediately insert a chest tube. Aggressive hemodynamic and respiratory resuscitation should be initiated.
- B. Tension pneumothorax should be treated immediately with a needle thoracostomy, followed by insertion of a chest tube.

II. Technique of chest tube insertion
- A. The patient should be placed in the supine position, with involved side elevated 10-20 degrees. The arm should be abducted at 90 degrees. The usual site of insertion is the anterior axillary line at the level of the fourth intercostal space (nipple line). Cleanse the skin with Betadine iodine solution and drape the field. The intrathoracic tube distance can be estimated by the distance between the lateral chest wall and the apex of the lung. The intrathoracic tube distance should be marked with a clamp.
- B. Infiltrate 1% lidocaine into the skin, subcutaneous tissues, intercostal muscles, periosteum, and pleura using a 25-gauge needle. Use a scalpel to make a transverse skin incision, 2 centimeters wide, located over the rib just inferior to the interspace where the tube will penetrate the chest wall.
- C. A Kelly clamp should be used to bluntly dissect a subcutaneous tunnel from the skin incision, extending just over the superior margin of the rib. The nerve, artery, and vein located just below each rib should be avoided.
- D. Bluntly dissect over the rib and penetrate the pleura with the clamp, and open the pleura 1 centimeter.
- E. With a gloved finger, explore the subcutaneous tunnel, and palpate the lung medially. Exclude possible abdominal penetration, and verify correct location within the pleural space, use a finger to remove any local pleural adhesions.
- F. Use the Kelly clamp to grasp the tip of the thoracostomy tube (36 F, Argyle, internal diameter 12 mm), and direct it into the pleural space in a posterior, superior direction for pneumothorax evacuation. Guide the tube into the pleural space until the last hole is inside the pleural space.
- G. Attach the tube to 20 cm H_2O of suction. Suture the tube to the skin of the chest wall using O silk. An untied, vertical, mattress suture may be placed to close the skin when the chest tube is removed in a few days.
- H. Apply Vaseline gauze, 4 x 4 gauze sponges, and elastic tape. Obtain a chest x-ray to verify correct tube placement and to evaluate re-expansion of the lung.

III. Indications for thoracotomy after trauma
- A. >1500 mL blood from chest tube on insertion.
- B. >200 mL blood/hour from chest tube thereafter (for 2-4 hours).
- C. Massive air leak such that lung will not re-expand after a properly placed and functioning chest tube has been inserted.

Tension Pneumothorax

I. **Clinical signs**
   A. Tension pneumothorax will manifest as severe hemodynamic and respiratory compromise, a contralaterally deviated trachea, and decreased or absent breath sounds on the involved side.
   B. Signs of tension pneumothorax may include hyperresonance to percussion on the affected side; jugular venous distention, and asymmetrical chest wall motion with respiration.
II. **Radiographic findings.** Loss of lung markings of ipsilateral side is commonly seen. Flattening or inversion of the ipsilateral hemidiaphragm and contralateral shifting of the mediastinum are usually present. Flattening of the cardiomediastinal contour, and spreading of the ribs on the ipsilateral side may be apparent.
III. **Acute management of tension pneumothorax.** Place a chest tube as described above. A temporary large-bore IV catheter may be inserted at the level of the second intercostal space at the mid-clavicular line into the pleural space, until the chest tube is placed.

Flail Chest

I. **Clinical evaluation**
   A. Flail chest occurs after two or more adjacent ribs become fractured in two locations. Flail chest usually occurs secondary to severe, blunt chest injury. The fractured ribs allow a rib segment, without bony continuity with the chest wall, to move freely during breathing. Hypoxia may result from underlying pulmonary contusion.
   B. Arterial blood gases should be measured if respiratory compromise is significant. If the fracture is in the left lower rib cage, splenic injury should be excluded with CT-scan.
II. **Management of flail chest**
   A. Aggressive pulmonary suctioning and close observation for any signs of respiratory insufficiency or hypoxemia are recommended. Endotracheal intubation and positive-pressure ventilation is indicated for significant cases of flail chest if oxygenation is inadequate. Associated injuries, such as pneumothorax and hemothorax, should be treated with tube thoracostomy.
   B. Pain control with epidural or intercostal blockade may eliminate the need for intubation. Intubation is required if there are significant injuries with massive pulmonary contusion or poor pulmonary reserve.
   C. If mechanical ventilation is required, the ventilator should be set to assist control mode to put the flail segment at rest for several days. Thereafter, a trial of low rate, intermittent, mandatory ventilation may be attempted to check for return of flail, prior to attempting extubation.

Massive Hemothorax

I. **Clinical evaluation**
   A. Massive hemothorax is defined as greater than 1500 mL of blood lost into the thoracic cavity. It most commonly occurs secondary to penetrating

injuries.
- B. Signs of massive hemothorax include absence of breath sounds and dullness to percussion on the ipsilateral side and signs of hypovolemic shock.

II. Management

- A. Volume deficit should be replaced. The chest cavity should be decompressed with a chest tube. Two large-bore intravenous lines or a central venous line should be inserted. A cardiothoracic surgeon should be consulted as soon as possible.
- B. A chest tube should be inserted. The site of insertion should be at the level of the fifth or sixth intercostal space, along the midaxillary line, ipsilateral to the hemothorax. The chest tube should be inserted in a location away from the injury.
- C. Penetrating wounds should be cleaned and closed. The wound should be covered with Vaseline impregnated gauze to decrease the likelihood of tension pneumothorax.
- D. A thoracotomy is indicated if blood loss continues through the chest tube at a rate greater than 200 mL/hr for 2-3 consecutive hours. If the site of wound penetration is medial to the nipple anteriorly or medial to the scapula posteriorly, it has a higher probability of being associated with injury to the myocardium and the great vessels. If the wound is below the fourth intercostal space, abdominal injury should be excluded.
- E. Consider tetanus prophylaxis and empirical antibiotic coverage.

Cardiac Tamponade

distension of neck veins
HypoTN
muffled ♡ sounds

I. Clinical evaluation

- A. Cardiac tamponade most commonly occurs secondary to penetrating injuries. Cardiac tamponade can also occur when a central line penetrates the wall of the right atrium.
- B. Cardiac tamponade is often manifested by Beck's triad of venous pressure elevation, drop in the arterial pressure, and muffled heart sounds.
- C. Other signs include hypovolemic shock, pulseless electrical activity (electromechanical dissociation), low voltage ECG, and enlarged cardiac silhouette on chest x-ray.
- D. Kussmaul's sign, rise in venous pressure with inspiration, may be present. Pulsus paradoxus or elevated venous pressure may be present.

II. Management

- A. Pericardiocentesis or placement of a pericardial window is indicated if the patient is unresponsive to fluid resuscitation measures for hypovolemic shock.
- B. All patients who have a positive pericardiocentesis (recovery of non-clotting blood) due to trauma require open thoracotomy with inspection of the myocardium and the great vessels. Cardiothoracic surgery should be consulted.
- C. Intravenous fluids or blood should be given as temporizing measures on the way to the operating room.
- D. Other causes of hemodynamic instability or electromechanical dissociation that may mimic cardiac tamponade include tension pneumothorax, massive pulmonary embolism, or hypovolemic shock.
- E. Subxiphoid pericardial window is an equally rapid and safer procedure

than pericardiocentesis if equipment and experienced surgical personnel are available.

Other Life-Threatening Trauma Emergencies

I. **Cardiac contusions**
   A. Arrhythmias are the most common consequence of cardiac contusions. Pump failure can also occur.
   B. **Treatment.** The patient should receive cardiac monitoring for 24 hours or longer if arrhythmias are present. If pump failure is suspected, cardiac function should be assessed with an echocardiogram or Swan Ganz catheter. Inotropic support should be provided.

II. **Pulmonary contusions**
   A. Pulmonary contusions are the most common potentially fatal chest injuries. Respiratory failure and hypoxemia may develop gradually over several hours. The clinical severity of hypoxia does not correlate well with chest x-ray, however, a contusion visible the initial CHEST X-RAY predicts a need for mechanical ventilation.
   B. If pulmonary compromise is mild and there is no other injury, patients can be managed without intubation.
   C. Treatment of severe contusions, especially with multiple injuries consists of intubation, positive pressure ventilation, and PEEP.

III. **Traumatic aortic transection**
   A. Diagnosis of traumatic aortic transection requires a high index of suspicion after severe chest trauma.
   B. The chest x-ray may show a widened mediastinum, obscured aortic knob, and a left pleural cap. The diagnostic standard remains aortogram, although transesophageal echocardiogram and spiral CT-scan are also useful. Management consists of immediate surgical repair.

IV. **Pelvic fracture**
   A. Fracture of the pelvis can produce exsanguinating hemorrhage. Diagnosis is by physical examination, plain x-ray films, and CT-scan.
   B. Hemorrhage is often difficult or impossible to control at laparotomy. Most bleeding is venous, and may be decreased by external fixation of the pelvis. Arterial bleeding sometimes occurs, and requires angiographic embolization.
   C. Pelvic fractures are often associated with abdominal injury. Diagnostic peritoneal lavage can be utilized to establish the presence of internal hemorrhage, although CT-scan is preferred. Associated bladder or urethral injuries are also common.

V. **Traumatic esophageal injuries**
   A. **Clinical evaluation**
      1. Esophageal injuries are usually caused by penetrating chest injuries, severe blunt trauma to the abdomen, nasogastric tube placement, endoscopy, or by repeated vomiting (Boerhaave's syndrome).
      2. After rupture, esophageal contents leak into the mediastinum, followed by immediate or delayed rupture into the pleural space (usually on left), with resulting empyema.
      3. A high index of suspicion is required in transthoracic penetrating injuries. Transmediastinal penetrating injuries mandate a search for great vessel, tracheobronchial, and esophageal injuries.
   B. **Treatment of esophageal injuries.** Surgical therapy consists of primary

surgical repair of the esophagus, with drainage, or esophageal diversion in the neck and a gastrostomy. Perforated tumors should be resected. Empiric broad spectrum antibiotic therapy should be initiated.

References: See page 113.

Burns

Bruce M. Achauer, MD

Over 50,000 people are hospitalized every year for burn injuries, and more than one million people are burned each year in the US. Burn injuries cause over 5000 deaths each year in the US.

I. Initial assessment
A. An evaluation of the Airway, Breathing, and Circulation (the ABCs) should receive first priority. The history should include the time, location and circumstances of the injury, where the patient was found, and their condition. Past medical and social history, current medication usage, drug allergies, and tetanus status should be rapidly determined.
B. Smoke inhalation causes more than 50% of fire-related deaths. Patients sustaining an inhalation injury may require aggressive airway intervention. Most injuries result from the inhalation of toxic smoke; however, superheated air may rarely cause direct thermal injury to the upper respiratory tract.
C. Patients who are breathing spontaneously and at risk for inhalation injury should be placed on high-flow humidified oxygen. Patients trapped in buildings or those caught in an explosion are at higher risk for inhalation injury. These patients may have facial burns, singeing of the eyebrows and nasal hair, pharyngeal burns, carbonaceous sputum, or impaired mentation. A change in voice quality, striderous respirations, or wheezing may be noted. The upper airway may be visualized by laryngoscopy, and the tracheobronchial tree should be evaluated by bronchoscopy. Chest radiography is not sensitive for detecting inhalation injury.
D. Patients who have suffered an inhalation injury are also at risk for carbon monoxide (CO) poisoning. The pulse oximeter is not accurate in patients with CO poisoning because only oxyhemoglobin and deoxyhemoglobin are detected. CO-oximetry measurements are necessary to confirm the diagnosis of CO poisoning. Patients exposed to CO should receive 100% oxygen using a nonrebreather face mask. Hyperbaric oxygen (HBO) therapy reduces the half-life of CO to 23 minutes.

II. Burn assessment
A. After completion of the primary survey, a secondary survey should assess the depth and total body surface area (TBSA) burned.
B. **First-degree burns** involve the epidermis layer of the skin, but not the dermal layer. These injuries are characterized by pain, erythema, and lack of blisters. First-degree burns are not considered in calculation of the TBSA burned.
C. **Second-degree burns** are subdivided into superficial and deep partial-thickness burns.
   1. **Superficial partial-thickness** burn injury involves the papillary dermis, containing pain-sensitive nerve endings. Blisters or bullae may be present, and the burns usually appear pink and moist.

2. **Deep partial-thickness** burn injury damages both the papillary and reticular dermis. These injuries may not be painful and often appear white or mottled pink.
D. **Full-thickness or third-degree burns** involve all layers of the epidermis and dermis. They appear white or charred. These burns usually are painless because of destruction of nerve endings, but the surrounding areas are extremely painful. Third-degree burns are treated with skin grafting to limit scarring.
E. **Fourth-degree burns** involve structures beneath the subcutaneous fat, including muscle and bone.
F. Estimation of total body surface area burn is based upon the "rule of nines."

Assessment of Percentage of Burn Area	
Head	9%
Anterior Torso	18%
Posterior Torso	18%
Each Leg	18%
Each Arm	9%
Genitalia/perineum	1%

Classification of Burns
Minor
• Less than 15% TBSA burns in adults or less than 10% TBSA burns in children or the elderly with less than 2% full-thickness injury
Moderate
• Partial- and full-thickness burns of 15-25% TBSA in young adults, 10-20% in children younger than 10 and adults older than 40 • Full-thickness burns less than 10% TBSA, not involving special care area.
Major Burns
• Greater than 25% TBSA burns in young adults or greater than 20% TBSA in children younger than 10 and adults older than 40. • Full-thickness burns of 10% or greater. All burns of special care areas that are likely to result in either functional or cosmetic impairment (ie, face, hands, ears, or perineum). • All burns complicated by inhalation injury, high-voltage electrical injury, or associated major trauma. High-risk patients include infants, the elderly, and patients with complicated medical problems.

III. Management of moderate to severe burns
A. Initial fluid resuscitation–The Parkland Formula
1. Initiation of fluid resuscitation should precede initial wound care. In adults, IV fluid resuscitation is usually necessary in second- or third-degree burns involving greater than 20% TBSA. In pediatric patients, fluid resuscitation should be initiated in all infants with burns of 10% or greater TBSA and in older children with burns greater than 15% or greater TBSA.
2. Two large-bore IV lines should be placed. Lactated Ringer's solution is the most commonly used fluid for burn resuscitation.
3. The Parkland formula is used to guide initial fluid resuscitation during the first 24 hours. The formula calls for 4 cc/kg/TBSA burn (second and third degree) of lactated Ringer's solution over the fast 24 hours. Half of the fluid should be administered over the first eight hours post burn, and the remaining half should be administered over the next 16 hours. The volume of fluid given is based on the time elapsed since the burn.
4. A urine output of 0.5-1.0 mL/kg/h should be maintained. Patients with significant burns should have a Foley catheter inserted in order to monitor urine output.

B. A nasogastric (NG) tube should be placed in patients with burns involving 20% or more TBSA in order to prevent gastric distention and emesis associated with a paralytic ileus.
C. Antibiotics is not generally recommended for initial management of burns but may be considered in the young child with suspected streptococcal infection.
D. Laboratory studies should include a complete blood count, electrolytes, serum glucose, BUN, and creatinine. Additional laboratory studies may include an ABG, CO HB level, urinalysis, urine myoglobin, coagulation studies, blood type and screen, toxicology screen, serum ethanol level, and serum protein. Patients with known heart disease or patients at risk for cardiac complications require a baseline ECG. A chest x-ray and other radiographs should be obtained as indicated.
E. Pain control. After completion of the primary and secondary survey, priority should be given to pain management. Morphine 0.1 mg/kg IV or meperidine (Demerol) 1-2 mg/kg IV should be used on an hourly basis.
F. Complications associated with eschar formation may occur in circumferential, deep partial- or full-thickness burns. Emergent escharotomy can relieve life- or limb-threatening constrictions caused by circumferential burns.
G. Tetanus toxoid (0.5 cc) should be administered as indicated. If the wound is >50% of the body surface area, 250 units of tetanus immune globulin should also be administered.
H. Burn center transfer. Most burn patients require only outpatient care. Most moderate burns and all major burns require hospitalization. Burns involving more than 15% of the total body surface area in adults, or more than 10% in children, should be transferred to a burn center. Patients with other severe injuries, extremes of age or inhalation injury should also be admitted to a burn center.

IV. Management of minor burns
A. Home wound care, pain medication, and active range-of-motion exercises should be prescribed. Some patients require physical therapy.
B. Tetanus status should be assessed. The burn wound should be cleansed with a mild soap and water or saline. Devitalized tissue or ruptured blisters

should be débrided using aseptic technique. Unruptured blisters should be left intact.
- C. Most outpatient burns are managed with closed dressings applied with topical antibiotics. A thin layer of sulfadiazine 1% (Silvadene) cream can be applied to a sterile gauze using a tongue blade, and then the gauze should be applied to the burn. Dressings are changed daily or twice daily and can be removed under running water.
- D. **Silver sulfadiazine** should be avoided in patients with allergies to sulfonamides, pregnant women approaching or at term, or in newborn infants during the first two months of life. Silvadene therapy may rarely cause a transient leukopenia and staining of sun-exposed skin.

References: See page 113.

Pulmonary Disorders

Charles F. Chandler, MD

Airway Management and Intubation

Orotracheal intubation:
 Endotracheal tube size (interior diameter):
  Women 7.0-9.0 mm
  Men 8.0 -10.0 mm

1. **Prepare functioning suction apparatus.** Have bag and mask apparatus setup with 100% oxygen; and ensure that the patient can be adequately bag ventilated and that suction apparatus is available.
2. **If sedation and/or paralysis is required**, consider rapid sequence induction as follows:
    -Fentanyl (Sublimaze) 50 mcg increments IV (1 mcg/kg) **with:**
    -Midazolam hydrochloride (Versed) 1 mg IV q2-3 min, max 0.1-0.15 mg/kg; 2-5 mg IV doses q1-4h prn **followed by:**
    -Succinylcholine (Anectine) 0.6-1.0 mg/kg, at appropriate intervals.
    Note: These drugs may cause vomiting; therefore, cricoid cartilage pressure should be applied during intubation (Sellick maneuver).
3. **Position the patient's head in "sniffing" position** with head flexed at neck and extended. If necessary elevate the head with a small pillow.
4. **Ventilate the patient** with a bag mask apparatus and hyperoxygenate with 100% oxygen.
5. **Hold endoscope handle with left hand,** and use right hand to open the patient's mouth. Insert blade along the right side of mouth to the base of tongue, and push the tongue to the left. If using curved blade, advance to the vallecula (superior to epiglottis), and lift anteriorly, being careful not to exert pressure on the teeth. If using a straight blade, place it beneath the epiglottis and lift anteriorly.
6. **Place endotracheal tube (ETT)** into right corner of mouth and pass it through the vocal cords; stop just after the cuff disappears behind the vocal cords. If unsuccessful after 30 seconds, stop and resume bag and mask ventilation before reattempting. If necessary, use stilette to maintain the shape of the ETT; remove stilette after intubation. Application of lubricant jelly at the balloon facilitates passage through the vocal cords.
7. **Inflate cuff with syringe**, keeping cuff pressure $\leq$20 cm H_2O and attach the tube to an Ambu bag or ventilator. Confirm bilateral, equal expansion of the chest and equal bilateral breath sounds. Auscultate the abdomen to confirm that the ETT is not in the esophagus. If there is any question about proper ETT location, repeat laryngoscopy with tube in place to be sure it is located endotracheal; remove tube immediately if there is any doubt about proper location. Secure the tube with tape and note centimeter mark at the mouth. Suction the oropharynx and trachea.
8. **Confirm proper tube placement with a chest X-ray.** The tip of the ETT should be between the carina and thoracic inlet, or level with the top of the aortic notch.

Ventilator Management

I. **Indications for Ventilatory Support:** Respirations >35, vital capacity <15 mL/kg, negative inspiratory force $\leq$-25, pO2 <60 on 50% O_2, pH <7.2, pCO_2 $\geq$55, severe hypercapnia, hypoxia, severe metabolic acidosis.

II. **Initiation of ventilatory support**

   A. **Intubation**
   1. Prepare suction apparatus, laryngoscope, endotracheal tube. Clear airway and place oral airway, then hyperventilate with bag and mask attached to high flow oxygen.
   2. Midazolam (Versed) 1-2 mg IV boluses until sedated. 2-5 mg IV doses q1-4h prn.
   3. Intubate, inflate cuff, ventilate with bag, auscultate chest, and suction trachea.

   B. **Initial orders.** FiO_2 = 100%, PEEP = 3-5 cm H_2O, assist control 8-14 breaths/min, tidal volume = 800 mL (10-15 mL/kg ideal body weight), set rate so that minute ventilation (VE) is approximately 10 L/min. Alternatively, use intermittent mandatory ventilation mode with tidal volume and rate to achieve near-total ventilatory support. Consider pressure support in addition to IMV at 5-15 cm H_2O.

   C. ABG should be obtained in 30 min, CHEST X-RAY for tube placement, measure cuff pressure q8h (maintain $\leq$20 mmHg), pulse oximeter, arterial line, or monitor end tidal CO_2. Maintain oxygen saturation >90-95%.

   D. **Ventilator management**
   1. **Decreased minute ventilation.** Evaluate patient and rule out complications (endotracheal tube malposition, cuff leak, excessive secretions, bronchospasms, pneumothorax, worsening pulmonary disease, sedative drugs, pulmonary infection). Readjust ventilator rate to maintain mechanically assisted minute ventilation of 10 L/min. If peak airway pressure (AWP) is >45 cm H_2O, decrease tidal volume to 7-8 mL/kg (with increase in rate if necessary) or decrease ventilator flow rate.
   2. **Arterial saturation $\geq$94% and pO_2 >100,** reduce FIO_2 (each 1% decrease in FIO_2 reduces pO_2 by 7 mmHg); once FIO_2 is <60%, PEEP may be reduced by increments of 2 cm H_2O until PEEP is 3-5 cm H_2O. Maintain O_2 saturation of $\geq$90% (pO_2 >60).
   3. **Arterial saturation <90% and pO_2 <60,** increase FIO_2 up to 60-100%, then consider increasing PEEP by increments of 3-5 cm H_2O (PEEP >10 requires a PA catheter). Add additional PEEP until oxygenation is adequate with an FIO_2 of <60%.
   4. **Excessively low pH,** (pH <7.33): Increase rate and/or tidal volume. Keep peak airway pressure <40-50 cm H_2O if possible.
   5. **Excessively high pH** (>7.48): Reduce rate and/or tidal volume to lessen hyperventilation. If patient is breathing rapidly above ventilator rate, sedate patient.
   6. **Patient "fighting" ventilator:** Consider intermittent mandatory ventilation or spontaneous intermittent mandatory ventilation mode, or add sedation with or without paralysis (exclude complications or other causes of agitation). Paralytic agents should not be used without concurrent amnesia and/or sedation.
   7. **Sedation**
      a. Midazolam (Versed) 0.05 mg/kg IVP x1, then 0.02-0.1 mg/kg/hr IV infusion. Titrate in increments of 25-50%.

b. Lorazepam (Ativan) 1-2 mg IV ql-2h pm sedation or 0.005 mg/kg IVP x1, then 0.025-0.2 mg/kg/hr IV infusion. Titrate in increments of 25-50%.
   c. Morphine sulfate 2-5 mg IV q5min, max dose 20-30 mg OR 0.03-0.05 mg/kg/h IV infusion (50-100 mg in 500 mL D5W) titrated OR
   d. Propofol (Diprivan): 50 mcg/kg bolus over 5 min. then 5-50 mcg/kg/min. Titrate in increments of 5 mcg/kg/min.
8. Paralysis
   a. Pancuronium (Pavulon) is the agent of choice in most settings. This agent should be avoided in patients with a history of asthma (causes mast cell degranulation) and heart disease (vagolytic). Load with 0.08 mg/kg, then start a continuous infusion of 0.02-0.03 mg/kg/hr.
   b. Vecuronium (Norcuron) is an analog of pancuronium that does not cause hypertension or mast cell degranulation. It is the agent of choice with cardiac disease or hemodynamic instability. However, it has the highest incidence of post-neuromuscular blockade paralysis. Load with 0.1 mg/kg, then start a continuous infusion of 0.06 mg/kg/hr.
   c. Cisatracurium (Nimbex) is an isomer of atracurium with less histamine release and hypotension. It has no hepatic or renal excretion. The dosage is 0.15 mg/kg IV, then 0.3 mcg/kg/min IV infusion; titrate between 0.5-1.0 mcg/kg/min.
   d. All patients on neuromuscular blocking agents should be continuously monitored for degree of blockade with a peripheral nerve stimulator to a train of four of 90-95%.
9. **Loss of tidal volume:** If a difference between the tidal volume setting and the delivered volume occurs, check for a leak in the ventilator or inspiratory line. Check for a poor seal between the endotracheal tube cuff or malposition of the cuff in the subglottic area. If a chest tube is present, check for air leak.
10. **Weaning from mechanical ventilation**
    a. Consider extubation in patients with cardiovascular stability, a high PaO_2/FiO_2 ratios (>200) on low PEEP, and those able to protect their airway.
    b. The most common weaning method is the daily trial of spontaneous breathing. While at the bedside, the patient is placed on CPAP and allowed to breath on his own. If the respiratory rate/tidal volume ratio is <100, patients are rested on the previous settings until the next day.
    c. If they fail the T-tube trial, or their respiratory rate to tidal volume ratio is >100, they are rested on the previous settings until the next day.

Epistaxis

Roger Crumley, MD

Almost all persons have experienced a nosebleed at some time, and most nosebleeds resolve without requiring medical attention. Prolonged epistaxis, however, can be life-threatening, especially in the elderly or debilitated.

48 Epistaxis

I. Pathophysiology
   A. **Anterior epistaxis**, in the anterior two thirds of the nose, is usually visible on the septum and is the most common type of epistaxis. The anterior portion of the septum has a rich vascular supply known as Kiesselbach's plexus or Little's area, and most epistaxis originates in this region. Anterior bleeding can often be stopped by pinching the cartilaginous part of the nose.
   B. **Posterior epistaxis** from the posterior third of the nose accounts for 10% of nosebleeds. Bleeding is profuse because of the larger vessels in that location. It usually occurs in older patients, who have fragile vessels because of hypertension, atherosclerosis, coagulopathies, or weakened tissue. Posterior bleeds require aggressive treatment and hospitalization.

II. Causes of epistaxis
   A. **Trauma.** Nose picking, nose blowing, or sneezing can tear or abrade the mucosa and cause bleeding. Other forms of trauma include nasal fracture and nasogastric and nasotracheal intubation.
   B. **Desiccation.** Cold, dry air and dry heat contribute to an increased incidence of epistaxis during the winter.
   C. **Irritation.** Upper respiratory infections, sinusitis, allergies, topical decongestants, and cocaine sniffing may cause bleeding.
   D. Less common causes of anterior epistaxis include Wegener's granulomatosis, mid-line destructive disease, tuberculosis, syphilis, and tumors. Epistaxis is exacerbated by coagulopathy, blood dyscrasia, thrombocytopenia, or anticoagulant medication (NSAIDs, warfarin), hepatic cirrhosis, and renal failure.
   E. **Hypertension** complicates active bleeding by promoting rigid arteries, and arteriosclerosis weakens vessels.

III. Clinical evaluation of epistaxis
   A. The airway, breathing and circulation should be maintained. Hemodynamic evaluation for tachycardia, hypotension, or light-headedness should be completed immediately. Hypovolemic patients should be resuscitated with fluids and packed red blood cells. Oxygen should be administered and intravenous access established. When inserting the intravenous line, it is convenient to obtain blood for complete blood count and, if clinically indicated, type and screen, coagulation profile, and electrolytes.
   B. After stabilization, the site, cause, and amount of bleeding should be determined. Most patients do not require resuscitation. Posterior epistaxis in an elderly and debilitated patient can be life-threatening.
   C. **Determine the side of bleeding.** Unilateral nose bleeding suggests anterior epistaxis in Kiesselbach's plexus. Bilateral bleeding suggests posterior epistaxis caused by overflow around the posterior septum.
   D. **Determine whether epistaxis is anterior or posterior:** When the patient is upright, blood drains primarily from the anterior part of the nose in anterior bleeding, or it drains from the nasopharynx in posterior bleeding.
   E. **Assess the duration** of the nosebleed and any inciting incident (eg, trauma). Swallowed blood from epistaxis may cause melena. Hypertension, bleeding disorders, diabetes, alcoholism, liver disease, pulmonary disease, cardiac disease and arteriosclerosis should be assessed.
   F. **Medications** including aspirin, NSAIDs, warfarin, nasal sprays, and oxygen via nasal cannula should be sought.
   G. **Blood tests.** Hematologic tests include CBC, platelet count, INR, partial

IV. Localization of the site of bleeding

A. **Sedation.** When sedation is required, midazolam (Versed), 1-2 mg IV in adults and 0.035-0.2 mg/kg IV in children is recommended; overmedication may threaten the cough reflex which protects the airway.

B. **Drape the patient**, and furnish an emesis basin. Keep the patient sitting upright or leaning forward. A gown, gloves, mask, and protective eyewear should be worn because patients may inadvertently cough blood.

C. **A nasal speculum** and a suction apparatus with a #10 Frazier tip are used to aspirate blood from the nose and oropharynx. A bright headlight should be used.

D. **Anesthesia and vasoconstriction:** A cotton-tipped applicator or cotton pledget is used to apply a topical anesthetic (eg, 1% tetracaine or 4% lidocaine) and a topical vasoconstrictor (eg, 1% ephedrine, 1% phenylephrine, or 0.05% oxymetazoline) to the entire nasal mucosa. If a bleeding site is observed, press the vasoconstrictor applicator directly to that site.

E. **Visualization of bleeding site**
1. The nasal speculum should be used to localize active bleeding. Kiesselbach's plexus and the inferior turbinate are the most frequent sites of bleeding.
2. Posterior bleeding may be located by applying suction; when the suction tip is at the site of bleeding, blood will no longer well up.

V. Management of hemorrhage

A. Anterior septal hemorrhage can sometimes be stopped by nose pinching alone and by having the patient sit upright. If bleeding continues, application of the topical anesthetic and vasoconstrictor may stop it.

B. **Cauterization**
1. Bleeding sites that can be visualized should be cauterized with silver nitrate sticks; they work best in a dry field.
2. The septum should not be cauterized bilaterally at the same level because cartilaginous necrosis and septal perforation may result.

C. **Hemostatic agents.** Application of a hemostatic material (eg, microfibrillar collagen or oxidized regenerated cellulose) to the bleeding site may be useful. These products do not require removal because they dissolve in the nose after several days. The patient should lubricate the nose regularly with saline nasal spray and to use bacitracin ointment tid.

D. **Packing.** Gauze packing or a sponge pack applied to the anterior portion of the nose may be used as a tamponade for uncontrolled bleeding sites. These packs stay in place for 5 days.

E. **Anterior nasal pack**
1. The pack consists of 72 inches of half-inch gauze impregnated with antibiotic ointment. Topical anesthesia is necessary.
2. Use the nasal speculum to open the vestibule vertically. With the bayonet forceps, grasp the gauze approximately 10 cm from the end; place layers along the floor of the nose all the way back to the nasopharynx.
3. **An oral broad-spectrum antibiotic**, such as cephalexin (Keflex), 500 mg orally every 6 hours, is given while the pack is in place to prevent secondary sinusitis or toxic shock syndrome. The pack is removed after 5 days.

F. Sponge pack
1. This dry, compressed sponge is lubricated with an antibiotic ointment, then placed into the nasal cavity.
2. Once moistened with blood or saline, the sponge expands, filling the nasal cavity and exerting gentle pressure on the bleeding site.

G. Posterior pack
1. Posterior bleeding requires a posterior pack, and the patient should be admitted to the hospital. The posterior pack requires a sphenopalatine block and topical anesthetic.
2. The posterior pack is made by sewing together two tonsil tampons with 0-silk, leaving two 8-inch tails, and lubricating the tampons with antibiotic ointment.
3. Place a tight anterior gauze pack, and tie the tails around one or two dental rolls to stabilize the tampons.

H. Balloon pack
1. An effective alternative to the tampon posterior pack is a 14-French, 30-mL balloon Foley catheter.
2. Use the same anesthetic as for the tampon posterior pack, and cover the balloon with antibiotic ointment, and insert it through the nostril until the tip can be seen in the nasopharynx.

References: See page 113.

Disorders of the Alimentary Tract

Russell A. Williams, MD
I. James Sarfeh, MD
S.E. Wilson, MD

Acute Abdomen

I. Clinical evaluation of abdominal pain
   A. Onset and duration of the pain
      1. The duration, acuity, and progression of pain should be assessed, and the exact location of maximal pain at onset and at present should be determined. The pain should be characterized as diffuse or localized. The time course of the pain should be characterized as either constant, intermittent, decreasing, or increasing.
      2. Acute exacerbation of longstanding pain suggests a complication of chronic disease, such as peptic ulcer disease, inflammatory bowel disease, or cancer. Sudden, intense pain often represents an intraabdominal catastrophe (eg, ruptured aneurysm, mesenteric infarction, or intestinal perforation). Colicky abdominal pain of intestinal or ureteral obstruction tends to have a gradual onset.
   B. Pain character
      1. **Intermittent pain** is associated with spasmodic increases in pressure within hollow organs.
      2. **Bowel ischemia** initially causes diffuse crampy pain due to spasmodic contractions of the bowel. The pain becomes constant and more intense with bowel necrosis, causing pain out of proportion to physical findings. A history of intestinal angina can be elicited in some patients.
      3. **Constant pain.** Biliary colic from cystic or common bile duct obstruction usually is constant. Chronic pancreatitis causes constant pain. Constant pain also suggests parietal peritoneal inflammation, mucosal inflammatory conditions, or neoplasms.
      4. **Appendicitis** initially causes intermittent periumbilical pain. Gradually the pain becomes constant in the right lower quadrant as peritoneal inflammation develops.
   C. Associated symptoms
      1. **Constitutional symptoms** (eg, fatigue, weight loss) suggests underlying chronic disease.
      2. Gastrointestinal symptoms
         a. **Anorexia**, nausea and vomiting are commonly associated with acute abdominal disorders. The frequency, character, and timing of these symptoms in relation to pain and time of the last flatus or stool should be determined.
         b. **Constipation, obstipation, crampy pain and distention** usually predominate in distal small-bowel and colonic obstruction. Paralytic ileus causes constipation and distention.
         c. **Diarrhea** is suggestive of gastroenteritis or colitis but may also be seen in partial small-bowel obstruction or fecal impaction.
         d. **Small amounts of bleeding** may accompany esophagitis, diverticulitis, inflammatory bowel disease, and left colon cancer. Right colon cancers usually present with occult blood loss. Severe

abdominal pain accompanied by melena or hematochezia suggests ischemic bowel.
  - **e. Jaundice** with abdominal pain usually is caused by biliary stones. Obstruction of the common bile duct by cancer may also cause pain and jaundice.
  3. **Urinary symptoms.** Urinary tract infections may cause pain in the lower abdomen (cystitis) or flanks (pyelonephritis). Urinary tract infections are characterized by dysuria, frequency, and cloudy urine.
  4. **Recent menstrual and sexual history** should be determined in women with acute abdominal pain.
     - **a. Menstrual cycle.** Lower abdominal pain and a missed or irregular menses in a young woman suggests ectopic pregnancy. Pelvic inflammatory disease tends to cause bilateral lower abdominal pain. Ovarian torsion may cause intense, acute pain and vomiting. Chronic pain at the onset of menses suggests endometriosis.
     - **b. Pregnancy.** Ectopic pregnancy occurs in the first trimester. Threatened abortion, ovarian torsion, or degeneration of a uterine fibroid also may cause acute pain in women.
- **D. Medications**
  1. **Nonsteroidal anti-inflammatory drugs** predispose to ulcer disease.
  2. **Antibiotic** therapy may obscure the signs of peritonitis. Patients with abdominal pain and diarrhea who have received antibiotics may have pseudomembranous colitis.
  3. **Anticoagulants.** Warfarin therapy predisposes to retroperitoneal or intramural intestinal hemorrhage.
  4. **Thiazide diuretics** may rarely cause pancreatitis.
- **E. Surgical history.** Small bowel obstruction is often caused by postoperative adhesions.

II. Physical examination

- **A. General appearance.** Peritonitis is suggested by shallow, rapid breathing and the patient often will lie still with knees flexed to minimize peritoneal stimulation. Patients may be pale or diaphoretic. Cachexia may indicate malignancy or chronic illness.
- **B. Fever** suggests an inflammatory or infectious etiology. Tachycardia and tachypnea may be caused by pain, hypovolemia, or sepsis. Hypothermia and hypotension often suggest an infectious process. Pneumonia and myocardial infarction may occasionally cause pain that is felt in the abdomen.
- **C. Abdominal examination**
  1. **Inspection.** Surgical scars should be noted. Distention suggests obstruction, ileus, or ascites. Venous engorgement of the abdominal wall suggests portal hypertension. Masses or peristaltic waves may be visible. Hemoperitoneum may cause bluish discoloration of the umbilicus (Cullen's sign). Retroperitoneal bleeding (eg, from hemorrhagic pancreatitis) can cause flank ecchymoses (Turner's sign).
  2. **Auscultation.** Borborygmi may be heard with obstruction. A quiet, rigid tender abdomen may occur with generalized peritonitis. A tender, pulsatile mass suggests an aortic aneurysm rupture.
  3. **Palpation**
     - **a.** Palpation should be gently started at a point remote from the pain. Muscle spasm, tympany or dullness, masses and hernias should be sought.
     - **b. Peritoneal signs.** Rigidity is caused by reflex spasm of the abdom-

inal wall musculature from underlying inflamed parietal peritoneum. Stretch and release of inflamed parietal peritoneum causes rebound tenderness.
- c. **Common signs**
  - (1) **Murphy's sign.** Inspiratory arrest from palpation in the right upper quadrant occurs when an inflamed gallbladder descends to meet the examiner's fingers.
  - (2) **Obturator sign.** Suprapubic tenderness on internal rotation of the hip joint with the knee and hip flexed results from inflammation adjacent to the obturator internus muscle.
  - (3) **Iliopsoas sign.** Extension of the hip elicits tenderness in inflammatory disorders of the retroperitoneum.
  - (4) **Rovsing's sign.** Referred, rebound tenderness in the left lower quadrant suggests appendicitis.
- D. **Rectal and pelvic examination**
  1. **Digital examination of the rectum** may detect cancer, fecal impaction, or pelvic appendicitis. Stool should be checked for gross or occult blood.
  2. **Pelvic examination.** Vaginal discharge should be noted and cultured. Masses and tenderness should be sought bimanually. Adnexal or cervical motion tenderness indicate pelvic inflammatory disease.

III. Laboratory evaluation

- A. **Leukocytosis** or a left shift on differential cell count are non-specific findings for infection. Leukopenia may be present in sepsis. The hematocrit can detect anemia due to occult blood loss from cancer. The hematocrit may be elevated with plasma volume deficits.
- B. **Electrolytes.** Metabolic alkalosis occurs after persistent vomiting. Metabolic acidosis occurs with severe hypovolemia or sepsis.
- C. **Urinalysis.** Bacteriuria, pyuria, or positive leukocyte esterase suggest urinary tract infection. Hematuria suggests urolithiasis.
- D. **Liver function tests.** High transaminases with mild to moderate elevations of alkaline phosphatase and bilirubin suggests acute hepatitis. High alkaline phosphatase and bilirubin and mild elevations of transaminases suggests biliary obstruction.
- E. **Pancreatic enzymes.** Elevated amylase and lipase indicates acute pancreatitis. Hyperamylasemia also may occur in bowel infarction and perforated ulcer.
- F. **Serum beta-human chorionic gonadotropin** is required in women of childbearing age with abdominal pain to exclude ectopic gestation.

IV. Radiography

- A. **Plain abdominal films**
  1. **Acute abdomen series** includes an upright PA chest, plain abdominal film ("flat plate"), upright film, and a left lateral decubitus view of the abdomen.
  2. **Bowel obstruction**
     - a. **Small bowel obstruction** may cause multiple air-fluid levels with dilated loops of small intestine, associated with minimal colonic gas.
     - b. **Colonic obstruction** causes colonic dilation which can be distinguished from small intestine by the presence of haustral markings and absence of valvulae conniventes.
  3. **Free air** is seen on the upright chest x-ray under the hemidiaphragms. Intestinal perforation is the most common cause of free air. A recent laparotomy may also cause free air.

4. **Stones and calcifications.** Ninety percent of urinary stones are radiopaque. Only 15% of gallstones are visible on plain film. A fecalith in the right lower quadrant may suggest appendicitis. Vascular calcification may be visible in abdominal aneurysm.
- B. **Ultrasonography** is useful for evaluation of biliary colic, cholecystitis, or female reproductive system disorders.
- C. **Computed tomography with or without oral and/or rectal contrast** may help in evaluating the acute abdomen in the following situations:
  1. Unobtainable or highly atypical history or physical examination
  2. History of intraabdominal cancer
  3. Abdominal pain and fever in the immediate postlaparotomy period
  4. Acute pain superimposed on a history of chronic abdominal complaints
  5. A stable patient with suspected leaking abdominal aneurysm

References: See page 113.

Appendicitis

About 10% of the population will develop acute appendicitis during their lifetime. The disorder most commonly develops in the teens and twenties. Appendicitis is caused by appendiceal obstruction, mucosal ischemia, infection, and perforation.

I. Diagnosis of appendicitis
A. **Clinical presentation.** Early appendicitis is characterized by progressive midabdominal discomfort, unrelieved by the passage of stool or flatus. Ninety percent of patients are anorexic, 70% have nausea and vomiting, and 10% have diarrhea. The pain migrates to the right lower quadrant after 4-6 hours. Peritoneal irritation is associated with pain on movement.
B. **Physical examination**
  1. Mild fever and tachycardia are common in appendicitis.
  2. Abdominal palpation should begin away from the right lower quadrant. Point tenderness over the right lower quadrant is the most definitive finding. Pain in the right lower quadrant during palpation of the left lower quadrant (Rovsing's sign) indicates peritoneal irritation. The degree of direct tenderness and rebound tenderness should be assessed. The degree of muscular resistance to palpation reflects the severity of inflammation. Cutaneous hyperesthesia often overlies the region of maximal tenderness.
  3. **Psoas sign.** With the patient lying on the left side, slow extension of the right hip causes local irritation and pain. A positive psoas sign indicates retroperitoneal inflammation.
  4. **Obturator sign.** With the patient supine, passive internally rotation of the flexed right hip causes hypogastric pain.
  5. **Rectal examination** should evaluate the presence of localized tenderness or an inflammatory mass in the pelvis.
  6. **Pelvic examination,** in women, should be completed to assess cervical motion tenderness and to evaluate the presence of adnexal tenderness.
  7. The appendix usually is found at McBurney's point (two-thirds of the distance from the umbilicus to the anterior superior iliac spine).
  8. Diarrhea, urinary frequency, pyuria, or microscopic hematuria may suggest a retrocecal appendix, causing irritation of adjacent structures.

- C. Laboratory evaluation
    1. **Leukocyte count** greater than 11,000 cells/ul with polymorphonuclear cell predominance is common in children and young adults.
    2. **Urinalysis** is abnormal in 25% of patients with appendicitis. Pyuria, albuminuria, and hematuria are common. Bacteria suggest urinary tract infection. Hematuria suggests urolithiasis.
    3. **Serum pregnancy test** should be performed in women of childbearing age. A positive test suggests an ectopic pregnancy.
- D. Radiologic evaluation
    1. **Abdominal x-rays.** An appendicolith can be seen in only one-third of children and one-fifth of adults with appendicitis. An appendiceal mass can indent the cecum, and tissue edema can cause loss of peritoneal fat planes around the psoas muscle and kidney.
    2. **Ultrasonography.** Findings associated with appendicitis include wall thickening, luminal distention, lack of compressibility, abscess formation, and free intraperitoneal fluid.

II. Differential diagnosis
- A. Gastrointestinal diseases
    1. **Gastroenteritis** is characterized by nausea, emesis prior to the onset of abdominal pain, malaise, fever, and poorly localized abdominal pain and tenderness. The WBC count is less frequently elevated.
    2. **Meckel's diverticulitis** may mimic appendicitis.
    3. **Perforated peptic ulcer disease, diverticulitis, and cholecystitis** can present similarly to appendicitis.
- B. Urologic diseases
    1. **Pyelonephritis** is associated with high fever, rigors, and costovertebral pain and tenderness. Diagnosis is confirmed by urinalysis.
    2. **Ureteral colic.** Renal stones cause flank pain radiating into the groin. Tenderness is usually minimal and hematuria is present. The intravenous pyelogram is diagnostic.
- C. Gynecologic diseases
    1. **Pelvic inflammatory disease (PID).** The onset of pain in PID usually occurs within 7 days of menstruation. Cervical motion tenderness, a white vaginal discharge, and bilateral adnexal tenderness suggest PID. Ultrasound can help distinguish PID from appendicitis.
    2. **Ectopic pregnancy.** A pregnancy test should be performed in all female patients of childbearing age presenting with abdominal pain. Ultrasonography is diagnostic.
    3. **Ovarian cysts** can cause sudden pain by enlarging or rupturing. The cysts are detected by transvaginal ultrasonography.
    4. **Ovarian torsion.** The ischemic ovary often can be palpated on bimanual pelvic examination. The diagnosis is confirmed by ultrasonography.

References: See page 113.

Appendectomy Surgical Technique

I. Preoperative preparation
- A. Intravenous isotonic fluid replacement should be initiated to achieve good urinary output and to correct electrolyte abnormalities. Nasogastric suction should be initiated if the patient is vomiting or if peritonitis is present.
- B. Fever is treated with acetaminophen. Broad-spectrum antibiotic coverage

Appendectomy Surgical Technique

is initiated preoperatively. Antibiotic therapy should cover gram-negative and anaerobic organisms (Cefotan or Zosyn).

II. Surgical technique

A. After induction of anesthesia, place an incision over any appendiceal mass if palpable. If no mass is present, make a transverse skin incision over McBurney's point, located two thirds of the way between the umbilicus and anterior superior iliac spine. A transverse incision allows easy extension medially for greater exposure. Diffuse peritonitis should be explored through a midline incision.

B. Incise the subcutaneous tissues in the line of the transverse incision, and incise the external oblique aponeurosis in the direction of its muscle fibers. Spread the muscle with a Peon hemostat.

C. Incise the internal oblique fascia and spread the incision in the direction of its fibers. Sharply incise the transversus abdominis muscle, transversalis fascia, and peritoneum. Note the presence and characteristics of peritoneal fluid, and send purulent fluid for Gram's stain and aerobic and anaerobic culture.

D. Identify the base of the cecum by the converging taeniae coli, and raise the cecum, exposing the base of the appendix. Hook an index finger around the appendix, and gently break down any adhesions to adjacent tissues. Use gauze packing to isolate the inflamed appendix, and stabilize the appendix with a Babcock forceps.

E. Apply two clamps to the mesoappendix, then divide the mesoappendix between the clamps, then firmly ligate below the clamps with 000 silk or polyglycolic acid sutures. Apply an encircling purse-string suture of 000 silk at the end of the cecum about 0.8 cm from the base of the appendix. Place a hemostat at the proximal base of the appendix, and crush the appendix. Remove the hemostat and reapply it to the appendix distal to the crush. Use an 0 chromic catgut suture to ligate the crushed area below the hemostat.

F. Transect the appendix against the clamp. Invert the stump into the cecum with the purse-string suture, and tie the purse-string suture, burying the stump. Irrigate the peritoneum with normal saline, and examine the mesoappendix and abdominal wall for hemostasis. Close the peritoneum with continuous 000 catgut suture.

G. Close the internal oblique and transversus abdominis with interrupted O chromic catgut. Close the external oblique as a separate layer. Close the skin and subcutaneous tissues. A soft rubber Penrose drain should be placed if perforation has occurred. It should be brought out through a stab incision in the lateral abdominal wall or through the lateral end of the incision.

H. If the appendix is normal on inspection (5-20% of explorations), it should be removed, and alternative diagnoses should be investigated. The cecum, sigmoid colon, and ileum should be inspected, and mesenteric lymphadenopathy should be sought. Ovaries and fallopian tubes should be inspected for PID, ruptured cysts, or ectopic pregnancy. Bilious peritoneal fluid suggests perforation of a peptic ulcer or the gallbladder.

III. Intravenous antibiotics

A. Antibiotic prophylaxis should include coverage for bowel flora, including aerobes and anaerobes. Cefotetan (Cefotan), 1 gm IV q12h, or piperacillin/tazobactam (Zosyn), 4.5 gm IV q6h, should be given before the operation and discontinued after two doses postoperatively.

B. If perforation has occurred, IV antibiotics should be continued for 5-10

Hernias

A hernia is an abnormal opening in the abdominal wall, with or without protrusion of an intraabdominal structure. A hernia develops in 5% of men during their lifetime. The most common groin hernia in males or females is the indirect inguinal hernia. Femoral hernias are more common in females than in males.

I. Inguinal hernias
  A. **Indirect hernia sacs** pass through the internal inguinal ring lateral to the inferior epigastric vessels and lie within the spermatic cord. Two-thirds of inguinal hernias are indirect
  B. **Direct hernias** occur when viscera protrude through a weak area in the posterior inguinal wall. The base of the hernia sac lies medial to the inferior epigastric vessels, through Hesselbach's triangle, which is formed by the inferior epigastric artery, the lateral edge of the rectus sheath, and the inguinal ligament.
  C. **Combined (pantaloon) hernias** occur when direct and indirect hernias occur simultaneously.
  D. **Sliding hernias** occur when part of the wall of the sac is formed by a viscera (bladder, colon). Richter's hernias occur when part of the bowel (rather than the entire circumference) becomes trapped. Only a "knuckle" of bowel enters the hernia sac.
  E. **Incarcerated hernias** cannot be reduced into the abdominal cavity. Strangulated hernias are hernias with incarcerated contents and a compromised blood supply; intense pain indicates intestinal ischemia.
  F. **Inguinal anatomy**
     1. **Layers of abdominal wall:** Skin, subcutaneous fat, Scarpa's fascia, external oblique, internal oblique, transversus abdominous, transversalis fascia, peritoneum.
     2. **Hesselbach's triangle:** A triangle formed by the lateral edge of rectus sheath, the inferior epigastric vessels, and the inguinal ligament.
     3. **Inguinal ligament:** Ligament running from anterior superior iliac spine to the pubic tubercle.
     4. **Lacunar ligament:** Reflection of inguinal ligament from the pubic tubercle onto the iliopectineal line of the pubic ramus.
     5. **Cooper's ligament:** Strong, fibrous band located on the iliopectineal line of the superior public ramus.
     6. **External inguinal ring:** Opening in the external oblique aponeurosis; the ring contains the ilioinguinal nerve and spermatic cord or round ligament.
     7. **Internal ring:** Bordered superiorly by internal oblique muscle and inferomedially by the inferior epigastric vessels and the transversalis fascia.
     8. **Processus vaginalis:** A diverticulum of peritoneum which descends with the testicle and lies adjacent to the spermatic cord. The processus vaginalis may enlarge to become the sac of an indirect inguinal hernia.
     9. **Femoral canal:** Formed by the borders of the inguinal ligament,

lacunar ligament, Cooper's ligament, and femoral sheath.
- **G. Clinical evaluation**
  1. **Inguinal hernias** usually present as an intermittent mass in the groin. The symptoms can usually be reproduced by a purposeful Valsalva maneuver. A bowel obstruction may rarely be the first manifestation of a hernia.
  2. **Physical examination.** An inguinal bulge with a smooth, rounded surface is usually palpable. The bulge may become larger with straining. The hernia sac can be assessed by invaginating the hemiscrotum with an index finger passed through the external inguinal ring.
  3. **Radiologic evaluation.** X-ray studies are not usually needed. Ultrasonography or CT scanning may be necessary to evaluate small hernias, particularly in the obese patient.
- **H. Differential diagnosis.** Inguinal hernias are distinguished from femoral hernias by the fact that femoral hernias originate below the inguinal ligament. Inguinal adenopathy, lipomas, dilatation of the saphenous vein, and psoas abscesses may present as inguinal masses.
- **I. Treatment**
  1. **Preoperative evaluation and preparation.** Hernias should be treated surgically. If incarceration or strangulation has occurred, broad-spectrum antibiotics and nasogastric suction should be initiated.
  2. **Reduction.** In uncomplicated cases, the hernia should be reduced by placing the patient in Trendelenburg's position or by gentle pressure applied over the hernia. Strangulated hernias should not be reduced because reduction may cause peritoneal contamination by a necrotic bowel loop and release of vasoactive agents from infarcted tissue.
  3. **Surgical repair**
     a. **Indirect inguinal hernias.** The aponeurosis of the external oblique muscle should be opened, then the cremaster muscle is opened, and the contents of the cord identified. The hernia sac is separated from the cord structures and transected. The neck should then be ligated, and the posterior abdominal wall should be repaired.
     b. **Direct inguinal hernias.** The external oblique should be opened and the cord structures should be separated from the hernia sac, then the sac should be inverted. The posterior abdominal wall is repaired by approximating the inferior arch of the transversus muscle (conjoint tendon) to the iliopubic tract (Bassini repair).
     c. **Lichtenstein (Tension-Free) Repair.** A mesh plug or patch is often used to produce a "tension free" repair.

II. Femoral hernias

- **A.** Femoral hernias account for 5% of all hernias, and 84% of femoral hernias occur in women. Incarceration or strangulation occur in 25% of femoral hernias.
- **B.** In femoral hernias, the abdominal viscera and peritoneum protrude through the femoral ring into the upper thigh. The femoral ring is limited medially by the lacunar ligament of Gimbernat, laterally by the femoral vein, anteriorly and proximally by the inguinal ligament, and posteriorly and distally by Cooper's ligament.
- **C. Clinical evaluation**
  1. Femoral hernias may present as a tender groin mass, and small-bowel obstruction may sometimes occur.
  2. **Physical examination.** The hernia sac manifests clinically as a mass

in the upper thigh, curving craniad over the inguinal region. It may appear while the patient is standing or straining and may disappear in the supine position.
    D. **Treatment.** A Cooper's ligament repair (McVey) through the inguinal approach is recommended.
III. **Abdominal wall hernias**
    A. **Incisional hernias** occur at sites of previous incisions. Hernias occur after 14% of abdominal operations.
    B. **Umbilical hernias** are congenital defects. Most newborn umbilical hernias close spontaneously by the second year of life. Patients with ascites have a high incidence of umbilical hernias.
    C. **Epigastric hernias** occur in the linea alba above the umbilicus.
    D. **Spigelian hernias** protrude near the termination of the transversus abdominis muscle at the lateral edge of the rectus abdominis muscle.
    E. **Lumbar hernias** occur superior to the iliac crest or below the last rib.
    F. **Obturator hernias** pass through the obturator foramen and present with bowel obstruction and focal tenderness on rectal examination.

Inguinal Hernia Repair Technique

I. **Indirect hernia**
    A. Prep and draped the skin of the abdomen, inguinal region, upper thigh, and external genitalia. Place the incision 1 cm above and parallel to the inguinal ligament. Begin the incision at a point just above, and medial to, the pubic tubercle, and extend it to a point two-thirds the distance to the anterior iliac spine. Incise the subcutaneous fat in the length of the incision down to the external oblique aponeurosis. Clear the external oblique muscle of overlying fat and identify the external inguinal ring. Incise the aponeurosis of the external oblique, beginning laterally and splitting the aponeurosis in the direction of its fibers, taking care not to injure the underlying ilioinguinal nerve. Expose the inguinal canal in which the spermatic cord and the indirect inguinal hernia are located.
    B. Use blunt dissection to mobilize the spermatic cord and the associated hernia up to the level of the pubic tubercle. Lift these structures up from the floor of the inguinal canal, and encircle with a Penrose drain. Retract the drain anteriorly, and free the remainder of the cord from the floor of the canal. Use sharp and blunt dissection to incise the anterior muscular and fascial investments of the cord.
    C. Sharply incise the internal spermatic fascia, and locate the hernial sac; identify the spermatic artery, venous plexus, and vas deferens before opening the sac.
    D. Incise the indirect hernial sac anteriorly along its long axis. Place an index finger inside the hernial sac, and separate the sac from surrounding cord structures, using sharp and blunt dissection. Carry the dissection proximally to the internal inguinal ring.
    E. Close the sac with a circumferential purse-string suture on an atraumatic, gastrointestinal needle. Tie this suture, being careful that no abdominal organs are within the purse string. Reinforce this ligation by placing another transfixion suture through the sac 1 mm distal to the purse-string suture. Transect the sac a few millimeters below the second suture, and cut both sutures and allow sac to retract into the retroperitoneum. Remove the sac. Inspect the floor of the inguinal canal. If there is only

60 Inguinal Hernia Repair Technique

minimal dilation of the internal ring, the hernia repair can be completed by placing a few interrupted sutures at the medial border of the internal ring and completing a Bassini repair.

- F. If the hernia is moderately sized, use a modification of the Bassini repair. Place a series of interrupted sutures in the transversalis fascia, beginning medially at the level of the pubic tubercle. Carry the sutures laterally as far as the medial border of the internal ring. Incorporate the posterior fibers of the conjoint tendon or use the posterior fascia of the transversalis abdominous muscle with some of the muscular fibers of the internal oblique muscle.
- G. Begin suturing medially at Cooper's ligament, and transition at the femoral sheath to Poupart's ligament. Place the sutures 1 cm apart, and use nonabsorbable monofilament 00 suture. Tie the sutures to reinforce the floor of the inguinal canal.
- H. Replace the ilioinguinal nerve and the spermatic cord in the inguinal canal, and reapproximate the external oblique aponeurosis over the cord with interrupted, nonabsorbable, 000 sutures.
- I. Close the subcutaneous tissues with interrupted, fine, absorbable sutures in Scarpa's fascia, and close the skin with staples or subcuticular sutures. Apply a sterile dressing.

II. Repair of direct inguinal hernias

- A. The skin incision is the same as for repair of the indirect inguinal hernia. The direct inguinal hernia appears as a diffuse bulge in the area of Hesselbach's triangle, appreciated by palpating with a fingertip. Reduce the direct inguinal hernia with a series of interrupted, inverting, 00, nonabsorbable sutures placed in the redundant preperitoneal tissue.
- B. The fascial defect in Hesselbach's triangle is repaired with a Cooper's ligament or modified McVay-type repair. Sharp and blunt dissection of the floor of the inferior portion of the inguinal canal should be used to expose the lacunar ligament and Cooper's ligament. Dissect laterally along Cooper's ligament as far as the medial aspect of the femoral vein. A relaxing incision should be made in the deep portion of the anterior rectus sheath, then grasp the medial and superior edge of the defect in Hesselbach's triangle with Allis clamps.
- C. A series of interrupted sutures is placed, beginning medially at the pubic tubercle, and carried laterally as far as the femoral vein. Check the appropriate snugness of the deep inguinal ring. When all sutures are placed, tie the sutures medial to lateral. Replace the cord and the ilioinguinal nerve in the bed of the inguinal canal, and reapproximate the external oblique aponeurosis over these structures.

III. Lichtenstein (Tension-Free) Repair

- A. One of the most commonly performed open herniorrhaphy techniques is the tension-free (Lichtenstein) repair. A tension-free hernioplasty performed with mesh reinforcement of the inguinal floor significantly decreases the recurrence rate.
- B. The Lichtenstein repair is routinely performed in an outpatient setting with local anesthesia. A Marlex mesh patch is sutured to the aponeurotic tissue overlying the pubic bone, with continuation of this suture along the edge of the inguinal (Poupart's) ligament to a point lateral to the internal inguinal ring.
- C. The lateral edge of the mesh is slit to allow passage of the spermatic cord between the split limbs of the mesh. The cephalad edge of the mesh is sutured to the conjoined tendon, with the internal oblique edge

overlapped by 2 cm. The two tails of the lateral aspect of the mesh are sutured together, incorporating the margin of the inguinal ligament.
References: See page 113.

Upper Gastrointestinal Bleeding

When bleeding is believed to be caused by a source proximal to the ligament of Treitz or the source of bleeding is indeterminant, flexible upper gastrointestinal endoscopy is indicated after initial resuscitation and stabilization.

I. Clinical evaluation
　A. Initial evaluation of upper GI bleeding should estimate the severity, duration, location, and cause of bleeding. A history of bleeding occurring after forceful vomiting suggests Mallory-Weiss Syndrome.
　B. Abdominal pain, melena, hematochezia (bright red blood per rectum), history of peptic ulcer, cirrhosis or prior bleeding episodes may be present.
　C. **Precipitating factors.** Use of aspirin, nonsteroidal anti-inflammatory drugs, alcohol, or anticoagulants should be sought.

II. Physical examination
　A. **General:** Pallor and shallow, rapid respirations may be present; tachycardia indicates a 10% blood volume loss. Postural hypotension (increase in pulse of 20 and a systolic blood pressure fall of 10-15 mmHg), indicates a 20-30% loss.
　B. **Skin:** Delayed capillary refill and stigmata of liver disease (jaundice, spider angiomas, parotid gland hypertrophy) should be sought.
　C. **Abdomen:** Scars, tenderness, masses, hepatomegaly, and dilated abdominal veins should be evaluated. Stool occult blood should be checked.

III. Laboratory evaluation:
CBC, SMA 12, liver function tests, amylase, INR/PTT, type and cross for pRBC, ECG.

IV. Differential diagnosis of upper bleeding:
Peptic ulcer, gastritis, esophageal varices, Mallory-Weiss tear, esophagitis, swallowed blood from epistaxis, malignancy (esophageal, gastric), angiodysplasias, aorto-enteric fistula, hematobilia.

V. Management of upper gastrointestinal bleeding
　A. If the bleeding appears to have stopped or has significantly slowed, medical therapy with H2 blockers and saline lavage is usually all that is required.
　B. Two 14- to16-gauge IV lines should be placed. Normal saline solution should be infused until blood is ready, then transfuse 2-6 units of pRBCs as fast as possible.
　C. A large bore nasogastric tube should be placed, followed by lavage with 2 L of room temperature tap water. The tube should then be connected to low intermittent suction, and the lavage should be repeated hourly. The NG tube may be removed when bleeding is no longer active.
　D. Oxygen is administered by nasal cannula. Urine output should be monitored.
　E. Serial hematocrits should be checked and maintained greater than 30%. Coagulopathy should be assessed and corrected with fresh frozen plasma, vitamin K, cryoprecipitate, and platelets.
　F. Definitive diagnosis requires upper endoscopy, at which time electrocoagulation, banding, and/or local injection of vasoconstrictors at

62 Upper Gastrointestinal Bleeding

bleeding sites may be completed. Surgical consultation should be requested in unstable patients or patients who require more than 6 units of pRBCs.

Clinical Indicators of Gastrointestinal Bleeding and Probable Source		
Clinical Indicator	Probability of Upper Gastrointestinal source	Probability of Lower Gastrointestinal Source
Hematemesis	Almost certain	Rare
Melena	Probable	Possible
Hematochezia	Possible	Probable
Blood-streaked stool	Rare	Almost certain
Occult blood in stool	Possible	Possible

VI. Peptic Ulcer Disease

A. Peptic ulcer disease is the commonest cause of upper gastrointestinal bleeding, responsible for 27-40% of all upper gastrointestinal bleeding episodes. Duodenal ulcer is more frequent than gastric ulcer. Three fourths of all peptic ulcer hemorrhages subside spontaneously.

B. Upper gastrointestinal endoscopy is the most effective diagnostic technique for peptic ulcer disease. Endoscopic therapy is the method of choice for controlling active ulcer hemorrhage.

C. Proton-pump inhibitor administration is effective in decreasing rebleeding rates with bleeding ulcers. Therapy consists of intravenous pantoprazole.

  1. **Pantoprazole (Protonix)** dosage is 80 mg IV, followed by continuous infusion with 8 mg/hr, then 40 mg PO bid when active bleeding has subsided.
  2. Twice daily dosing of oral proton pump inhibitors may be a reasonable alternative when intravenous formulations are not available. Oral omeprazole (Prilosec) for duodenal ulcer: 20 mg qd for 4-8 weeks. Gastric ulcers: 20 mg bid. Lansoprazole (Prevacid), 15 mg qd. Esomeprazole (Nexium) 20-40 mg qd.

D. Indications for surgical operation include (1) severe hemorrhage unresponsive to initial resuscitative measures; (2) failure of endoscopic or other nonsurgical therapies; and (3) perforation, obstruction, or suspicion of malignancy.

E. Duodenal ulcer hemorrhage. Suture ligation of the ulcer-associated bleeding artery combined with a vagotomy is indicated for duodenal ulcer hemorrhage that does not respond to medical therapy. Truncal vagotomy and pyloroplasty is widely used because it is rapidly and easily accomplished.

F. Gastric ulcer hemorrhage is most often managed by truncal vagotomy and pyloroplasty with wedge excision of ulcer.

G. Transcatheter angiographic embolization of the bleeding artery responsible for ulcer hemorrhage is recommended in patients who fail endoscopic attempts at control and who are poor surgical candidates.

VII. Hemorrhagic Gastritis
- **A.** The diffuse mucosal inflammation of gastritis rarely manifest as severe or life-threatening hemorrhage. Hemorrhagic gastritis accounts for 4% of upper gastrointestinal hemorrhage. The bleeding is usually mild and self-limited. When coagulopathy accompanies cirrhosis and portal hypertension, however, gastric mucosal bleeding can be brisk and refractory.
- **B.** Endoscopic therapy can be effective for multiple punctate bleeding sites, but when diffuse mucosal hemorrhage is present, selective intra-arterial infusion of vasopressin may control bleeding. For the rare case in which surgical intervention is required, total gastrectomy is the most effective procedure.

VIII. Mallory-Weiss syndrome
- **A.** This disorder is defined as a mucosal tear at the gastroesophageal junction following forceful retching and vomiting.
- **B.** Treatment is supportive, and the majority of patients stop bleeding spontaneously. Endoscopic coagulation or operative suturing may rarely be necessary.

References: See page 113.

Esophageal Varices

Esophageal varices eventually develop in most patients with cirrhosis, but variceal bleeding occurs in only one third of them. The initiating event in the development of portal hypertension is increased resistance to portal outflow.

Causes of Portal Hypertension

Presinusoidal
    Extrahepatic causes
    Portal vein thrombosis
    Extrinsic compression of the portal vein
    Cavernous transformation of the portal vein
    Intrahepatic causes
    Sarcoidosis
    Primary biliary cirrhosis
    Hepatoportal sclerosis
    Schistosomiasis
Sinusoidal: Cirrhosis, alcoholic hepatitis
Postsinusoidal
    Budd-Chiari syndrome (hepatic vein thrombosis)
    Veno-occlusive disease
    Severe congestive heart failure
    Restrictive heart disease

I. Pathophysiology
- **A.** Varices develop annually in 5% to 15% of patients with cirrhosis, and varices enlarge by 4% to 10% each year. Each episode of variceal hemorrhage carries a 20% to 30% risk of death.
- **B.** After an acute variceal hemorrhage, bleeding resolves spontaneously in 50% of patients. Bleeding is least likely to stop in patients with large varices and a Child-Pugh class C cirrhotic liver.

64 Esophageal Varices

II. Management of variceal hemorrhage

A. Primary prophylaxis
1. All patients with cirrhosis should undergo endoscopy to screen for varices every 2 to 3 years.
2. Propranolol (Inderal) and nadolol (Corgard) reduce portal pressure through beta, blockade. Beta-blockade reduces the risk of bleeding by 45% and bleeding-related death by 50%. The beta-blocker dose is adjusted to decrease the resting heart rate by 25% from its baseline, but not to less than 55 to 60 beats/min.
3. Propranolol (Inderal) is given at 10 to 480 mg daily, in divided doses, or nadolol (Corgard) 40 to 320 mg daily in a single dose.

B. Treatment of acute hemorrhage
1. Variceal bleeding should be considered in any patient who presents with significant upper gastrointestinal bleeding. Signs of cirrhosis may include spider angiomas, palmar erythema, leukonychia, clubbing, parotid enlargement, and Dupuytren's contracture. Jaundice, lower extremity edema and ascites are indicative of decompensated liver disease.
2. The severity of the bleeding episode can be assessed on the basis of orthostatic changes (eg, resting tachycardia, postural hypotension), which indicates one-third or more of blood volume loss.
3. Blood should be replaced as soon as possible. While blood for transfusion is being made available, intravascular volume should be replenished with normal saline solution. Once euvolemia is established, the intravenous infusion should be changed to solutions with a lower sodium content (5% dextrose with 1/2 or 1/4 normal saline). Blood should be transfused to maintain a hematocrit of at least 30%. Serial hematocrit estimations should be obtained during continued bleeding.
4. Fresh frozen plasma is administered to patients who have been given massive transfusions. Each 3 units of PRBC should be accompanied by $CaCL_2$ 1 gm IV over 30 min. Clotting factors should be assessed. Platelet transfusions are reserved for counts below 50,000/mL in an actively bleeding patient.
5. If the patient's sensorium is altered because of hepatic encephalopathy, the risk of aspiration mandates endotracheal intubation. Placement of a large-caliber nasogastric tube (22 F or 24 F) permits tap water lavage for removal of blood and clots in preparation for endoscopy.
6. **Octreotide acetate (Sandostatin)** is a synthetic, analogue of somatostatin, which causes splanchnic vasoconstriction. Octreotide is the drug of choice in the pharmacologic management of acute variceal bleeding. Octreotide infusion should be started with a loading dose of 50 micrograms, followed by an infusion of 50 micrograms/hr. Treatment is continued until hemorrhage subsides. Definitive endoscopic therapy is performed shortly after hemostasis is achieved.
7. **Endoscopic therapy**
   a. A sclerosant (eg, morrhuate [Scleromate]) is injected into each varix. Complications include bleeding ulcers, dysphagia due to strictures, and pleural effusions.
   b. Endoscopic variceal ligation with elastic bands is an alternative to sclerotherapy because of fewer complications and similar efficacy.
   c. If bleeding persists (or recurs within 48 hours of the initial episode) despite pharmacologic therapy and two endoscopic therapeutic

attempts at least 24 hours apart, patients should be considered for salvage therapy with TIPS or surgical treatment (transection of esophageal varices and devascularization of the stomach, portacaval shunt, or liver transplantation).
8. **Transjugular intrahepatic portosystemic shunt (TIPS)** consists of the angiographic creation of a shunt between hepatic and portal veins which is kept open by a fenestrated metal stent. It decompresses the portal system, controlling active variceal bleeding over 90% of the time. Complications include secondary bleeding, worsening encephalopathy in 20%, and stent thrombosis or stenosis.

C. **Secondary prophylaxis**
1. A patient who has survived an episode of variceal hemorrhage has an overall risk of rebleeding that approaches 70% at 1 year.
2. **Endoscopic sclerotherapy** decreases the risk of rebleeding (50% versus 70%) and death (30% to 60% versus 50% to 75%). Endoscopic variceal ligation is superior to sclerotherapy. Banding is carried out every 2 to 3 weeks until obliteration.

References: See page 113.

Helicobacter Pylori Infection and Peptic Ulcer Disease

The spiral-shaped, gram-negative bacterium *Helicobacter pylori* is found in gastric mucosa or adherent to the lining of the stomach. Acute infection is most commonly asymptomatic but may be associated with epigastric burning, abdominal distention or bloating, belching, nausea, flatulence, and halitosis. *H. pylori* infection can lead to ulceration of the gastric mucosa and duodenum and is associated with malignancies of the stomach. The prevalence of *H. pylori* infection is as high as 52 percent.

I. Pathophysiology
A. Helicobacter pylori (HP), a spiral-shaped, flagellated organism, is the most frequent cause of peptic ulcer disease (PUD). Nonsteroidal anti-inflammatory drugs (NSAIDs) and pathologically high acid-secreting states (Zollinger-Ellison syndrome) are less common causes. More than 90% of ulcers are associated with H. pylori. Eradication of the organism cures and prevents relapses of gastroduodenal ulcers.
B. **Complications of peptic ulcer disease** include bleeding, duodenal or gastric perforation, and gastric outlet obstruction (due to inflammation or strictures).

II. Clinical evaluation
A. **Symptoms of PUD** include recurrent upper abdominal pain and discomfort. The pain of duodenal ulceration is often relieved by food and antacids and worsened when the stomach is empty (eg, at nighttime). In gastric ulceration, the pain may be exacerbated by eating.
B. Nausea and vomiting are common in PUD. Hematemesis ("coffee ground" emesis) or melena (black tarry stools) are indicative of bleeding.
C. **Physical examination.** Tenderness to deep palpation is often present in the epigastrium, and the stool is often guaiac-positive.

Peptic Ulcer Disease

Presentation of Uncomplicated Peptic Ulcer Disease

Epigastric pain (burning, vague abdominal discomfort, nausea)
  Often nocturnal
  Occurs with hunger or hours after meals
  Usually temporarily relieved by meals or antacids
  Persistence or recurrence over months to years
  History of self-medication and intermittent relief

   D. NSAID-related gastrointestinal complications. NSAID use and *H pylori* infection are independent risk factors for peptic ulcer disease. The risk is 5 to 20 times higher in persons who use NSAIDs than in the general population. Misoprostol (Cytotec) has been shown to prevent both NSAID ulcers and related complications. The minimum effective dosage is 200 micrograms twice daily; total daily doses of 600 micrograms or 800 micrograms are significantly more effective.

III. When to test and treat

   A. In the absence of alarm symptoms for cancer or complicated ulcer disease, the approach to testing in patients with dyspepsia can be divided into four clinical scenarios: (1) known peptic ulcer disease, currently or previously documented; (2) known nonulcer dyspepsia; (3) undifferentiated dyspepsia, and (4) gastroesophageal reflux disease (GERD).

   B. Peptic ulcer disease. Treatment of *H. pylori* infection in patients with ulcers almost always cures the disease and reduces the risk for perforation or bleeding.

   C. Nonulcer disease. There is no convincing evidence that empiric eradication of *H. pylori* in patients with nonulcer dyspepsia improves symptoms.

   D. Undifferentiated dyspepsia. A test-and-treat strategy is recommended in which patients with dyspepsia are tested for the presence of *H. pylori* with serology and treated with eradication therapy if the results are positive. Endoscopy is reserved for use in patients with alarm signs or those with persistent symptoms despite empiric therapy.

Alarm Signs for Risk of Gastric Cancer of Complicated Ulcer Disease

Older Than 45 years	Abdominal mass
Rectal bleeding or melena	Jaundice
Weight los of >10 percent of body weight	Family history of gastric cancer
Anemia	Previous history of peptic ulcer
Dysphagia	Anorexia/early satiety

Evaluation for Helicobacter pylori-Related Disease

Clinical scenario	Recommended test
Dyspepsia in patient with alarm symptoms for cancer or complicated ulcer (eg, bleeding, perforation)	Promptly refer to a gastroenterologist for endoscopy.
Known PUD, uncomplicated	Serology antibody test; treat if result is positive.
Dyspepsia in patient with previous history of PUD not previously treated with eradication therapy	Serology antibody test; treat if result is positive.
Dyspepsia in patient with PUD previously treated for *H. pylori*	Stool antigen or urea breath test; if positive, treat with regimen different from the one previously used; retest to confirm eradication. Consider endoscopy.
Undifferentiated dyspepsia (without endoscopy)	Serology antibody test; treat if result is positive.
Documented nonulcer dyspepsia (after endoscopy)	Unnecessary
GERD	Unnecessary
Asymptomatic with history of documented PUD not previously treated with eradication therapy	Serology antibody test; treat if result is positive.
Asymptomatic	Screening unnecessary

E. Gastroesophageal Reflux Disease. *H. pylori* infection does not increase the risk of GERD. Eradication therapy does not eliminate GERD symptoms (sensation of burning and regurgitation).

IV. *Helicobacter pylori* Tests

A. Once testing and eradication are chosen, several diagnostic tests are available. Unless endoscopy is planned, a practical approach is to use serology to identify initial infection, and use the stool antigen test or urea breath test to determine cure, if indicated.

Noninvasive Testing Options for Detecting Helicobacter pylori

Test	What does it measure?	Sensitivity	Test of cure?	Comments
Serology: laboratory-based ELISA	IgG	90 to 93	No	Accurate; convenient for initial infection; titers may remain positive after one year

Test	What does it measure?	Sensitivity	Test of cure?	Comments
Whole blood: office-based ELISA	IgG	50 to 85	No	Less accurate but fast, convenient
Stool: HpSA	H. pylori antigens	95 to 98	Yes	Relatively convenient and available
Urea breath test	Urease activity	95 to 100	Yes	Sensitivity reduced by acid suppression

- B. **Endoscopy and Biopsy.** Alarm symptoms for cancer or ulcer complication warrant prompt endoscopic evaluation. A gastric antral biopsy specimens is considered the gold standard for detecting the presence of H. pylori. Cultures of biopsy specimens obtained during endoscopy can be tested for antimicrobial resistance in cases of treatment failure.
- C. **Serology/ELISA.** When endoscopy is not performed, the most commonly used diagnostic approach is the laboratory-based serologic antibody test. This enzyme-linked immunosorbent assay (ELISA) detects IgG antibodies to H. pylori, indicating current or past infection. A positive serologic test suggests active infection in patients who have not undergone eradication therapy. The serologic test results may not revert to negative once the organism is eradicated; therefore, the test is not used to identify persistent infection.
- D. **Stool testing with enzyme-linked immunoassay** for H. pylori antigen in stool specimens is highly sensitive and specific, the stool antigen test reverts to negative from five days to a few months after eradication of the organism, with 90 percent specificity. This test is useful in confirming eradication, and, because it is office-based, is less costly and more convenient than the urea breath test. False-positive results may occur even four weeks following eradication therapy.
- E. **Urea Breath Test.** The urea breath test is a reliable test for cure and can detect the presence or absence of active H. pylori infection with greater accuracy than the serologic test. It is usually administered in the hospital outpatient setting because it requires time and special equipment.

V. **Principles of treatment**
- A. Antimicrobial resistance and incomplete treatment are major reasons for treatment failure. Continued therapy for 14 days is the most reliable and effective regimen.

Helicobacter Pylori Infection and Peptic Ulcer Disease

Triple Therapy Regimens for *Helicobacter pylori* Infection

Treatment (10 to 14 days of therapy recommended)	Convenience factor	Tolerability
1. Omeprazole (Prilosec), 20 mg two times daily *or* Lansoprazole (Prevacid), 30 mg two times daily *plus* Metronidazole (Flagyl), 500 mg two times daily *or* Amoxicillin, 1 g two times daily *plus* Clarithromycin (Biaxin), 500 mg two times daily **Prepackaged triple-therapy(Prevpac):** taken bid for 14 days; consists of 30 mg lansoprazole, 1 g amoxicillin, and 500 mg clarithromycin.	Twice-daily dosing	Fewer significant side effects, but more abnormal taste versus other regimens
2. Ranitidine bismuth citrate (Tritec), 400 mg twice daily *plus* Clarithromycin, 500 mg twice daily *or* Metronidazole, 500 mg twice daily *plus* Tetracycline, 500 mg twice daily *or* Amoxicillin, 1 g twice daily 92 (RMA)	Twice-daily dosing	Increased diarrhea versus other regimens

B. Triple and quadruple therapies have eradication rates approaching 90 percent or more.

C. Post-Treatment Followup
1. Routine laboratory testing for cure is not required in patients whose symptoms respond to eradication therapy.
2. Routine, noninvasive follow-up testing also can be considered in patients who have persistent symptoms following eradication therapy. In these patients, the stool antigen test, performed four weeks following therapy, is a convenient method. Patients with a history of ulcer complications, gastric mucosa-associated lymphoid tissue (MALT), or early gastric cancer should undergo a routine post-treatment urea breath test or endoscopy to ensure successful eradication.

D. Treatment of NSAID-related ulcers
1. When the ulcer is caused by NSAID use, healing of the ulcer is greatly facilitated by discontinuing the NSAID. Acid antisecretory therapy with an H2-blocker or proton pump inhibitor speeds ulcer healing. Proton pump inhibitors are more effective in inhibiting gastric acid production and are often used to heal ulcers in patients who require continuing NSAID treatment.
2. If serologic or endoscopic testing for H pylori is positive, antibiotic treatment is necessary.
3. **Acute H_2-blocker therapy**
   a. **Ranitidine (Zantac)**, 150 mg bid or 300 mg qhs.
   b. **Famotidine (Pepcid)**, 20 mg bid or 40 mg qhs.
   c. **Nizatidine (Axid Pulvules)**, 150 mg bid or 300 mg qhs.
   d. **Cimetidine (Tagamet)**, 400 mg bid or 800 mg qhs.

70 Lower Gastrointestinal Bleeding

4. **Proton pump inhibitors**
   a. **Omeprazole (Prilosec)**, 20 mg qd.
   b. **Lansoprazole (Prevacid)**, 15 mg before breakfast qd.
   c. **Esomeprazole (Nexium)** 20-40 mg qd.
   d. **Pantoprazole (Protonix)** 40 mg PO, 20 minuted before the first meal of the day or IV once daily.
   e. **Rabeprazole (Aciphex)** 20 mg/day, 20 to 30 minutes before the first meal of the day.

VI. **Surgical treatment of peptic ulcer disease**
   A. **Indications for surgery** include exsanguinating hemorrhage, >5 units transfusion in 24 hours, rebleeding during same hospitalization, intractability, perforation, gastric outlet obstruction, and endoscopic signs of rebleeding.
   B. Unstable patients should receive a truncal vagotomy, oversewing of bleeding ulcer bed, and pyloroplasty.

References: See page 113.

Lower Gastrointestinal Bleeding

The spontaneous remission rates for lower gastrointestinal bleeding is 80 percent. No source of bleeding can be identified in 12 percent of patients, and bleeding is recurrent in 25 percent. Bleeding has usually ceased by the time the patient presents to the emergency room.

I. **Clinical evaluation**
   A. The severity of blood loss and hemodynamic status should be assessed immediately. Initial management consists of resuscitation with crystalloid solutions (lactated Ringers) and blood products if necessary.
   B. The duration and quantity of bleeding should be assessed; however, the duration of bleeding is often underestimated.
   C. **Risk factors** that may have contributed to the bleeding include nonsteroidal anti-inflammatory drugs, anticoagulants, colonic diverticulitis, renal failure, coagulopathy, colonic polyps, and hemorrhoids. Patients may have a prior history of hemorrhoids, diverticulosis, inflammatory bowel disease, peptic ulcer, gastritis, cirrhosis, or esophageal varices.
   D. **Hematochezia.** Bright red or maroon output per rectum suggests a lower GI source; however, 12 to 20% of patients with an upper GI bleed may have hematochezia as a result of rapid blood loss.
   E. **Melena.** Sticky, black, foul-smelling stools suggest a source proximal to the ligament of Treitz, but Melena can also result from bleeding in the small intestine or proximal colon.
   F. **Clinical findings**
      1. **Abdominal pain** may result from ischemic bowel, inflammatory bowel disease, or a ruptured aneurysm.
      2. **Painless massive bleeding** suggests vascular bleeding from diverticula, angiodysplasia, or hemorrhoids.
      3. **Bloody diarrhea** suggests inflammatory bowel disease or an infectious origin.
      4. **Bleeding with rectal pain** is seen with anal fissures, hemorrhoids, and rectal ulcers.
      5. **Chronic constipation** suggests hemorrhoidal bleeding. New onset of constipation or thin stools suggests a left sided colonic malignancy.

6. **Blood on the toilet paper** or dripping into the toilet water suggests a perianal source of bleeding, such as hemorrhoids or an anal fissure.
7. **Blood coating** the outside of stools suggests a lesion in the anal canal.
8. **Blood streaking** or mixed in with the stool may results from polyps or a malignancy in the descending colon.
9. **Maroon colored stools** often indicate small bowel and proximal colon bleeding.

II. Physical examination
   A. **Postural hypotension** indicates a 20% blood volume loss, whereas, overt signs of shock (pallor, hypotension, tachycardia) indicates a 30 to 40 percent blood loss.
   B. **The skin** may be cool and pale with delayed refill if bleeding has been significant.
   C. **Stigmata of liver disease**, including jaundice, caput medusae, gynecomastia and palmar erythema, should be sought because patients with these findings frequently have GI bleeding.

III. Differential diagnosis of lower GI bleeding
   A. **Angiodysplasia** and diverticular disease of the right colon accounts for the vast majority of episodes of acute lower GI bleeding. Most acute lower GI bleeding originates from the colon however 15 to 20 percent of episodes arise from the small intestine and the upper GI tract.
   B. **Elderly patients.** Diverticulosis and angiodysplasia are the most common causes of lower GI bleeding.
   C. **Younger patients.** Hemorrhoids, anal fissures and inflammatory bowel disease are most common causes of lower GI bleeding.

Clinical Indicators of Gastrointestinal Bleeding and Probable Source		
Clinical Indicator	**Probability of Upper Gastrointestinal source**	**Probability of Lower Gastrointestinal Source**
Hematemesis	Almost certain	Rare
Melena	Probable	Possible
Hematochezia	Possible	Probable
Blood-streaked stool	Rare	Almost certain
Occult blood in stool	Possible	Possible

IV. Diagnosis and management of lower gastrointestinal bleeding
   A. **Rapid clinical evaluation and resuscitation** should precede diagnostic studies. Intravenous fluids (1 to 2 liters) should be infused over 10- 20 minutes to restore intravascular volume, and blood should be transfused if there is rapid ongoing blood loss or if hypotension or tachycardia are present. Coagulopathy is corrected with fresh frozen plasma, platelets, and cryoprecipitate.
   B. When small amounts of bright red blood are passed per rectum, then lower GI tract can be assumed to be the source. In patients with large volume maroon stools, nasogastric tube aspiration should be performed to exclude massive upper gastrointestinal hemorrhage.
   C. If the nasogastric aspirate contains no blood then anoscopy and

sigmoidoscopy should be performed to determine weather a colonic mucosal abnormality (ischemic or infectious colitis) or hemorrhoids might be the cause of bleeding.
- D. **Colonoscopy** in a patient with massive lower GI bleeding is often nondiagnostic, but it can detect ulcerative colitis, antibiotic-associated colitis, or ischemic colon.
- E. **Polyethylene glycol-electrolyte solution** (CoLyte or GoLytely) should be administered by means of a nasogastric tube (Four liters of solution is given over a 2-3 hour period), allowing for diagnostic and therapeutic colonoscopy.

V. Definitive management of lower gastrointestinal bleeding

- A. **Colonoscopy**
  1. Colonoscopy is the procedure of choice for diagnosing colonic causes of GI bleeding. It should be performed after adequate preparation of the bowel. If the bowel cannot be adequately prepared because of persistent, acute bleeding, a bleeding scan or angiography is preferable.
  2. If colonoscopy fails to reveal the source of the bleeding, the patient should be observed because, in 80% of cases, bleeding ceases spontaneously.
- B. **Radionuclide scan or bleeding scan.** Technetium- labeled (tagged) red blood cell bleeding scans can detect bleeding sites when bleeding is intermittent. Localization may not he a precise enough to allow segmental colon resection.
- C. **Angiography**. Selective mesenteric angiography detects arterial bleeding that occurs at rates of 0.5 mL/per minute or faster. Diverticular bleeding causes pooling of contrast medium within a diverticulum. Bleeding angiodysplastic lesions appear as abnormal vasculature. When active bleeding is seen with diverticular disease or angiodysplasia, selective arterial infusion of vasopressin may be effective.
- D. **Surgery**
  1. If bleeding continues and no source can be found, surgical intervention is usually warranted. Surgical resection may be indicated for patients with recurrent diverticular bleeding, or for patients who have had persistent bleeding from colonic angiodysplasia and have required blood transfusions.
  2. Surgical management of lower gastrointestinal bleeding is ideally undertaken with a secure knowledge of the location and cause of the bleeding lesion. A segmental bowel resection to include the lesion and followed by a primary anastomosis is usually safe and appropriate in all but the most unstable patients.

VI. Diverticulosis

- A. Diverticulosis of the colon is present in more than 50% of the population by age 60 years. Bleeding from diverticula is relatively rare, affecting only 4% to 17% of patients at risk.
- B. In most cases, bleeding ceases spontaneously, but in 10% to 20% of cases, the bleeding continues. The risk of rebleeding after an episode of bleeding is 25%. Right-sided colonic diverticula occur less frequently than left-sided or sigmoid diverticula but are responsible for a disproportionate incidence of diverticular bleeding.
- C. Operative management of diverticular bleeding is indicated when bleeding continues and is not amenable to angiographic or endoscopic therapy. It also should be considered in patients with recurrent bleeding in the same colonic segment. The operation usually consists of a segmental bowel

resection (usually a right colectomy or sigmoid colectomy) followed by a primary anastomosis.

VII. Arteriovenous malformations

A. AVMs or angiodysplasias are vascular lesions that occur primarily in the distal ileum, cecum, and ascending colon of elderly patients. The arteriographic criteria for identification of an AVM include a cluster of small arteries, visualization of a vascular tuft, and early and prolonged filling of the draining vein.

B. The typical pattern of bleeding of an AVM is recurrent and episodic, with most individual bleeding episodes being self-limited. Anemia is frequent, and continued massive bleeding is distinctly uncommon. After nondiagnostic colonoscopy, enteroscopy should be considered.

C. Endoscopic therapy for AVMs may include heater probe, laser, bipolar electrocoagulation, or argon beam coagulation. Operative management is usually reserved for patients with continued bleeding, anemia, repetitive transfusion requirements, and failure of endoscopic management. Surgical management consists of segmental bowel resection with primary anastomosis.

VIII. Inflammatory bowel disease

A. Ulcerative colitis and, less frequently, Crohn's colitis or enteritis may present with major or massive lower gastrointestinal bleeding. Infectious colitis can also manifest with bleeding, although it is rarely massive.

B. When the bleeding is minor to moderate, therapy directed at the inflammatory condition is appropriate. When the bleeding is major and causes hemodynamic instability, surgical intervention is usually required. When operative intervention is indicated, the patient is explored through a midline laparotomy, and a total abdominal colectomy with end ileostomy and oversewing of the distal rectal stump is the preferred procedure.

IX. Tumors of the colon and rectum

A. Colon and rectal tumors account for 5% to 10% of all hospitalizations for lower gastrointestinal bleeding. Visible bleeding from a benign colonic or rectal polyp is distinctly unusual. Major or massive hemorrhage rarely is caused by a colorectal neoplasm; however, chronic bleeding is common. When the neoplasm is in the right colon, bleeding is often occult and manifests as weakness or anemia.

B. More distal neoplasms are often initially confused with hemorrhoidal bleeding. For this reason, the treatment of hemorrhoids should always be preceded by flexible sigmoidoscopy in patients older than age 40 or 50 years. In younger patients, treatment of hemorrhoids without further investigation may be appropriate if there are no risk factors for neoplasm, there is a consistent clinical history, and there is anoscopic evidence of recent bleeding from enlarged internal hemorrhoids.

X. Anorectal disease

A. When bleeding occurs only with bowel movements and is visible on the toilet tissue or the surface of the stool, it is designated *outlet bleeding*. Outlet bleeding is most often associated with internal hemorrhoids or anal fissures.

B. Anal fissures are most commonly seen in young patients and are associated with severe pain during and after defecation. Other benign anorectal bleeding sources are proctitis secondary to inflammatory bowel disease, infection, or radiation injury. Additionally, stercoral ulcers can develop in patients with chronic constipation.

C. Surgery for anorectal problems is typically undertaken only after failure of

XI. Ischemic colitis
A. Ischemic colitis is seen in elderly patients with known vascular disease. The abdomen pain may be postprandial and associated with bloody diarrhea or rectal bleeding. Severe blood loss is unusual but can occur.
B. Abdominal films may reveal "thumb-printing" caused by submucosal edema. Colonoscopy reveals a well-demarcated area of hyperemia, edema and mucosal ulcerations. The splenic flexure and descending colon are the most common sites. Most episodes resolve spontaneously, however, vascular bypass or resection may be required.

References: See page 113.

Anorectal Disorders

I. Hemorrhoids
A. Hemorrhoids are dilated veins located beneath the lining of the anal canal. Internal hemorrhoids are located in the upper anal canal. External hemorrhoids are located in the lower anal canal.
B. The most common symptom of internal hemorrhoids is painless rectal bleeding, which is usually bright red and ranges from a few drops to a spattering stream at the end of defecation. If internal hemorrhoids remain prolapsed, a dull aching may occur. Blood and mucus stains may appear on underwear, and itching in the perianal region is common.

Classification of Internal Hemorrhoids		
Grade	Description	Symptoms
1	Non-prolapsing	Minimal bleeding
2	Prolapse with straining, reduce when spontaneously prolapsed	Bleeding, discomfort, pruritus
3	Prolapse with straining, manual reduction required when prolapsed	Bleeding, discomfort, pruritus
4	Cannot be reduced when prolapsed	Bleeding, discomfort, pruritus

C. **Management of internal hemorrhoids**
  1. **Grade 1 and uncomplicated grade 2 hemorrhoids** are treated with dietary modification (increased fiber and fluids).
  2. **Symptomatic grade 2 and grade 3 hemorrhoids.** Treatment consists of hemorrhoid banding with an anoscope. Major complications are rare and consist of excessive pain, bleeding, and infection. Surgical hemorrhoidectomy may sometimes be necessary.
  3. **Grade 4 hemorrhoids** require surgical hemorrhoidectomy.
D. **External hemorrhoids**
  1. External hemorrhoids occur most often in young and middle-aged adults, becoming symptomatic only when they become thrombosed.

2. External hemorrhoids are characterized by rapid onset of constant burning or throbbing pain, accompanying a new rectal lump. Bluish skin-covered lumps are visible at the anal verge.
3. **Management of external hemorrhoids**
   a. If patients are seen in the first 48 hours, the entire lesion can be excised in the office. Local anesthetic is infiltrated, and the thrombus and overlying skin are excised with scissors. The resulting wound heals by secondary intention.
   b. If thrombosis occurred more than 48 hours prior, spontaneous resolution should be permitted to occur.

II. Anal fissures

A. An anal fissure is a longitudinal tear in the distal anal canal, usually in the posterior or anterior midline. Patients with anal fissures complain of perirectal pain which is sharp, searing or burning and is associated with defecation. Bleeding from anal fissures is bright red and not mixed with the stool.

B. Anal fissures may be associated with secondary changes such as a sentinel tag, hypertrophied anal papilla, induration of the edge of the fissure, and anal stenosis. Crohn's disease should be considered if the patient has multiple fissures, or whose fissure is not in the midline.

C. Anal fissures are caused by spasm of the internal anal sphincter. Risk factors include a low-fiber diet and previous anal surgery.

D. **Treatment of anal fissures**
   1. High-fiber foods, warm sitz baths, stool softeners (if necessary), and daily application of 1% hydrocortisone cream to the fissure should be initiated. These simple measures may heal acute anal fissures within 3 weeks in 90% of patients.
   2. **Lateral partial internal sphincterotomy** is indicated when 4 weeks of medical therapy fails. The procedure consists of surgical division of a portion of the internal sphincter, and it is highly effective. Adverse effects include incontinence to flatus and stool.

III. Levator ani syndrome and proctalgia fugax

A. Levator ani syndrome refers to chronic or recurrent rectal pain, with episodes lasting 20 minutes or longer. Proctalgia fugax is characterized by anal or rectal pain, lasting for seconds to minutes and then disappearing for days to months.

B. Levator ani syndrome and proctalgia fugax are more common in patients under age 45, and psychological factors are not always present.

C. Levator ani syndrome is caused by chronic tension of the levator muscle. Proctalgia fugax is caused by rectal muscle spasm. Stressful events may trigger attacks of proctalgia fugax and levator ani syndrome.

D. **Diagnosis and clinical features**
   1. Levator ani syndrome is characterized by a vague, indefinite rectal discomfort or pain. The pain is felt high in the rectum and is sometimes associated with a sensation of pressure.
   2. Proctalgia fugax causes pain that is brief and self limited. Patients with proctalgia fugax complain of sudden onset of intense, sharp, stabbing or cramping pain in the anorectum.
   3. In patients with levator ani syndrome, palpation of the levator muscle during digital rectal examination usually reproduces the pain.

E. **Treatment**
   1. **Levator ani syndrome.** Treatment with hot baths, nonsteroidal anti-inflammatory drugs, muscle relaxants, or levator muscle massage is

recommended. EMG-based biofeedback may provide improvement in pain.
  2. **Proctalgia fugax.** For patients with frequent attacks, physical modalities such as hot packs or direct anal pressure with a finger or closed fist may alleviate the pain. Diltiazem and clonidine may provided relief.

IV. Pruritus ani
  A. Pruritus ani is characterized by the intense desire to scratch the skin around the anal orifice. It occurs in 1% of the population. Pruritus ani may be related to fecal leakage.
  B. Patients report an escalating pattern of itching and scratching in the perianal region. These symptoms may be worse at night. Anal hygiene and dietary habits, fecal soiling, and associated medical conditions should be sought.
  C. Examination reveals perianal maceration, erythema, excoriation, and lichenification. A digital rectal examination and anoscopy should be performed to assess the sphincter tone and look for secondary causes of pruritus. Patients who fail to respond to 3 or 4 weeks of conservative treatment should undergo further investigations such as skin biopsy and sigmoidoscopy or colonoscopy.
  D. **Treatment and patient education**
   1. Patients should clean the perianal area with water following defecation, but avoid soaps and vigorous rubbing. Following this, the patient should dry the anus with a hair dryer or by patting gently with cotton. Between bowel movements a thin cotton pledget dusted with unscented cornstarch should be placed against the anus. A high fiber diet is recommended to regulate bowel movements and absorb excess liquid. All foods and beverages that exacerbate the itching should be eliminated.
   2. Topical medications are not recommended because they may cause further irritation. If used, a bland cream such as zinc oxide or 1% hydrocortisone cream should be applied sparingly two to three times a day.
   3. Diphenhydramine (Benadryl) or hydroxyzine (Vistaril) may relieve the itching and allow the patient to sleep.

V. Perianal abscess
  A. The anal glands, located in the base of the anal crypts at the level of the dentate line, are the most common source of perianal infection. Acute infection causes an abscess, and chronic infection results in a fistula.
  B. The most common symptoms of perianal abscess are swelling and pain. Fevers and chills may occur. Perianal abscess is common in diabetic and immunosuppressed patients, and there is often a history of chronic constipation. A tender mass with fluctuant characteristics or induration is apparent on rectal exam.
  C. **Management of perianal abscess**. Perianal abscesses are treated with incision and drainage using a local anesthetic. Large abscesses require regional or general anesthesia. A cruciate incision is made close to the anal verge and the corners are excised to create an elliptical opening which promotes drainage. An antibiotic, such as Zosyn, Timentin, or Cefotetan, is administered.
  D. About half of patients with anorectal abscesses will develop a fistula tract between the anal glands and the perianal mucosa, known as a fistula-in-ano. This complication manifests as either incomplete healing of the

drainage site or recurrence. Healing of a fistula-in-ano requires a surgical fistulotomy.

Fistula-in-Ano

A fistula-in-ano develops when an anorectal abscess forms a fistula between the anal canal and the perianal skin. The fistula may develop after an anorectal abscess has been drained operatively, or the fistula may develop spontaneously.

I. **Clinical evaluation**
   A. The fistula is characterized by persistent purulent or feculent drainage, soiling the underwear.
   B. The fistula orifice can be seen just outside the anal verge. Complex fistulae may have multiple tracts with multiple orifices.

II. **Treatment of fistula-in-ano**
   A. Fistulae will not resolve without definitive treatment. The more common type of fistula, located at the anorectal junction, has an external opening where it can be drained operatively. The entire epithelialized tract must be found and obliterated.
   B. Goodsall's rule predicts the course of fistulae that exit the skin within 3 cm of the anal verge. Anterior fistulae go straight toward the anorectal junction; posterior fistulae curve toward the posterior midline and enter the anorectal junction.
   C. A pilonidal cyst-sinus (coccygeal region) can be difficult to distinguish from a fistula-in-ano. Probing the tract under anesthesia usually will reveal its origin.
   D. **Fistulotomy.** For fistulae that do not cross both internal and external sphincters, the tract should be unroofed and curetted. The lesion should then be allowed to heal by secondary intention.
   E. **Fistulectomy.** Deeper fistulae should be treated by coring out the epithelialized tract to its origin. The fistula may recur.
   F. **Seton procedure.** Complex fistulae or fistulae that traverse the sphincter can be treated by looping a heavy suture through the entire tract under tension. The suture should be tightened weekly until it "cuts" gradually to the surface. The tract will heal gradually behind the suture.

Colorectal Cancer

Charles Theuer, MD

Colorectal cancer is the second most common solid malignancy in adults and the second leading cause of cancer death in the US.

I. **Clinical evaluation of colorectal cancer**
   A. Flexible sigmoidoscopy is indicated for screening of asymptomatic, healthy adults over age 50. All adults with anemia or guaiac positive stools should be evaluated for colorectal cancer; older adults (>40) should be evaluated even if other sources of bleeding have been found. Hemorrhoids and cancer can coexist.

78 Colorectal Cancer

- **B.** Flexible sigmoidoscopy plus air contrast barium enema is adequate to evaluate the colon when the source of bleeding is thought to be benign anorectal disease. Total colonoscopy should be performed for any adult with gross or occult rectal bleeding and no apparent anorectal source.
- **C.** Left-sided or rectal lesions are characterized by blood streaked stools, change in caliber or consistency of stools, obstipation, alternating diarrhea and constipation, and tenesmus.
- **D.** Right-sided lesions are characterized by a triad of iron deficiency anemia, right lower quadrant mass, and weakness. Cancers occasionally present as a large bowel obstruction, perforation or abscess.

II. Laboratory evaluation

- **A.** Complete blood count with indices will often reveal a hypochromic, microcytic anemia. Liver function tests may sometimes be elevated in metastatic disease.
- **B. Carcinoembryonic antigen (CEA)** may be elevated in colorectal cancer, but it is a nonspecific test which may also be elevated in other malignancies, inflammatory bowel disease, cigarette smokers, and some normal persons. CEA is valuable in monitoring the response to treatment and as a marker for recurrence or metastases, requiring adjuvant therapy. It should be measured prior to resection of the tumor and at intervals postoperatively.
- **C.** Colorectal cancer is detected by colonoscopy with biopsies. Barium enema may complement colonoscopy since BE shows the exact anatomic location of the tumor. A chest X-ray should be done to search for metastases to the lungs. A CT scan should be done in cases where liver function test are elevated.

III. Management of colorectal carcinoma

- **A.** Surgical resection is indicated for colorectal adenocarcinoma, regardless of stage. Resection of the primary lesion prevents obstruction or perforation.
- **B.** Extremely advanced rectal lesions, which are not resectable, may be candidates for palliative radiation and a diverting colostomy.
- **C.** The extent of resection is determined by the relationship of the lesion to the lymphatic drainage and blood supply of the colon.
    1. **Cecum or right colon.** Right hemicolectomy.
    2. **Hepatic flexure.** Extended right hemicolectomy.
    3. **Mid-transverse colon:** Transverse colectomy or extended left or right hemicolectomy.
    4. **Splenic flexure or left colon.** Left hemicolectomy.
    5. **Sigmoid colon.** Sigmoid colectomy.
    6. **Upper or middle rectum.** Low anterior rectosigmoid resection with primary anastomosis.
    7. **Lower rectum.** Abdominoperineal resection with permanent, end-colostomy or local excision.
- **D. Preoperative bowel preparation**
    1. Mechanical cleansing of the lumen, followed by decontamination with nonabsorbable oral antibiotics decreases the chance of infectious complications and allows for primary anastomosis. Fully obstructed patients cannot be prepped and must have a temporary colostomy.
    2. Polyethylene glycol solution (CoLyte or GoLYTELY) is usually administered as 4 liters over 4 hours on the day before surgery. Oral phospho-soda (given as two 1 1/2 ounce doses in 8 ounces of water) can be substituted for polyethylene glycol in patients with normal renal

function. The Nichols-Condon prep consists of 1 g neomycin sulfate and 1 g erythromycin base PO at 2:00, 3:00 and 11:00 pm the day before operation. Cefotetan is given 1-2 gm IV 30 minutes before operation.

    3. Patients with middle and lower rectal tumors should be staged with endoanal ultrasound. Tumors that invade through the muscularis propria (T3) or involve lymph nodes (N1) should be offered neoadjuvant therapy with radiation therapy and 5-fluorouracil.

  E. Adjuvant chemotherapy is recommended for advanced colon lesions with the addition of pelvic radiation for advanced rectal tumors. Adjuvant therapy is reserved for locally advanced lesions (B2) or those with metastases to regional lymph nodes or distant organs (C1, C2, D).

  F. Pathologic staging of the tumor is done postoperatively by histologic examination of the surgical specimen.

IV. Staging of colorectal carcinoma

  A. **Astler-Coller modification of Dukes' Classification**

    Stage A: Limited to mucosa and submucosa. Nodes negative.

    Stage B1: Extends into, but not through, muscularis propria; nodes negative.

    Stage B2: Extends through muscularis propria; nodes negative.

    Stage C1: Same as B1, except nodes positive.

    Stage C2: Same as B2, except nodes positive.

V. Management of obstructing carcinomas of the left colon

  A. Correct fluid deficits and electrolyte abnormalities. Nasogastric suction is useful, but it is not adequate to decompress the acutely obstructed colon.

  B. The Hartmann procedure is indicated for distal descending and sigmoid colon lesions. This procedure consists of resection of the obstructing cancer and formation of an end-colostomy and blind rectal pouch. The colostomy can be taken down and anastomosed to the rectal pouch at a later date.

  C. Primary resection with temporary end-colostomy and mucous fistula should be done for lesions of the transverse and proximal descending colon. This procedure consists of resection of the obstructing cancer and creation of a functioning end-colostomy and a defunctionalized distal limb with separate stomas. The colostomy can be taken down and continuity restored at a later date.

  D. An emergency decompressive loop colostomy can be considered for acutely ill patients. After four to six weeks, a hemicolectomy can be completed. A primary anastomosis may be done in selected patients with a prepared bowel.

VI. Management of obstructing carcinomas of the ascending colon.
Correct fluid deficits, electrolyte abnormalities, and initiate nasogastric suction. A right hemicolectomy with primary anastomosis of the terminal ileum to the transverse colon can be performed on most patients. A temporary ileostomy is rarely needed.

References: See page 113.

Mesenteric Ischemia

Mesenteric ischemia is classified as acute mesenteric ischemia (AMI) and chronic mesenteric ischemia (CMI). AMI is subdivided into occlusive and nonocclusive mesenteric ischemia. Occlusive mesenteric ischemia results from either thrombotic or embolic arterial or venous occlusion.

Approximately 80% of cases of AMI are occlusive in etiology, with arterial emboli or thromboses in 65% of cases and venous thrombosis in 15%. Arterial occlusions result from emboli in 75% of patients and in situ thrombosis cause the remaining 25%. Nonocclusive mesenteric ischemia is caused by low perfusion states and is responsible for 20% of AMI.

I. Clinical evaluation
A. Mesenteric arterial embolism
1. The median age of patients presenting with mesenteric arterial embolism is 70 years. The overwhelming majority of emboli lodge in the superior mesenteric artery (SMA). Emboli originating in the left atrium or ventricle are the most common cause of SMA embolism.
2. Risk factors include advanced age, coronary artery disease, cardiac valvular disease, history of dysrhythmias, atrial fibrillation, post-myocardial infarction mural thrombi, history of thromboembolic events, aortic surgery, aortography, coronary angiography, and aortic dissection. A previous history of peripheral emboli is present in 20%.
3. The disorder usually presents as sudden onset of severe poorly localized periumbilical pain, associated with nausea, vomiting, and frequent bowel movements. Pain is usually out of proportion to the physical findings and may be the only presenting symptom.
4. The abdomen may be soft with only mild tenderness. Absent bowel sounds, abdominal distension or guarding are indicative of severe disease.
5. Blood in the rectum is present in 16% of patients, and occult blood is present in 25% of patients. Peritoneal signs develop when the ischemic process becomes transmural.

B. Mesenteric arterial thrombosis
1. Thrombosis usually occurs in the area of atherosclerotic narrowing in the proximal SMA. The proximal jejunum through the distal transverse colon becomes ischemic.
2. SMA thrombosis usually occurs in patients with chronic, severe, visceral atherosclerosis. A history of abdominal pain after meals is present in 20-50% of patients. Patients are often elderly, with coronary artery disease, severe peripheral vascular disease, or hypertension.
3. SMA thrombosis presents with gradual onset of abdominal pain and distension. A history of postprandial abdominal pain and weight loss is present in half of cases. Pain is usually out of proportion to the physical findings, and nausea and vomiting are common.
4. Signs of peripheral vascular disease, such as carotid, femoral or abdominal bruits, or decreased peripheral pulses are frequent. Abdominal distension, absent bowel sounds, guarding, rebound and localized tenderness, and rigidity indicate advanced bowel necrosis.

II. Diagnostic evaluation of acute mesenteric ischemia
A. Leukocyte count is elevated in most cases of mesenteric ischemia. In patients with SMA emboli, 42% have a metabolic acidosis. The serum amylase is elevated in half of patients.

- **B. Plain radiography.** Abdominal and chest x-rays help to exclude the presence of free air or bowel obstruction. In rare instances, plain films of the abdomen reveal signs of ischemic bowel such as pneumatosis intestinalis, portal venous gas, or a thickened bowel wall with thumbprinting. However, plain films will be normal in the majority of cases.
- **C. Angiography** is the gold standard for the diagnosis of AMI and is also used for therapeutic infusion of the vasodilator, papaverine. After obtaining plain abdominal films to rule out the presence of free air or obstruction, angiography must be obtained, especially in those patients in whom there is a strong clinical suspicion for AMI.

III. Emergency management
- **A. Stabilization and initial management**
    1. Patients with significant hypotension require rapid fluid resuscitation, and vasopressors may be used.
    2. If hemoglobin is low, blood should be given. Patients who appear acutely ill should receive parenteral antibiotics to cover for gram-negative enteric bacteria as well as anaerobes after blood cultures are drawn.
- **B. Papaverine**
    1. Intraarterial infusion of papaverine into the superior mesenteric artery will increase mesenteric perfusion by relieving mesenteric vasoconstriction.
    2. Papaverine is started at angiography and continued postoperatively if laparotomy is performed. The dosing is 60 mg IV bolus, followed by a 30-60 mg/h continuous infusion at a concentration of 1 mg/mL. Papaverine improves survival by 20-50%.
- **C. Acute mesenteric infarction with embolism**
    1. Once embolism is confirmed at angiography, papaverine infusion is started, then laparotomy should be performed to evaluate bowel viability. Surgical intervention may involve arteriotomy with embolectomy and bowel resection if nonviable necrotic bowel is found. Postoperative anticoagulation is recommended for all patients.
    2. Patients without peritoneal signs with minor emboli, who achieve pain relief with vasodilator infusion, may be managed nonoperatively with repeated angiograms.
- **D. Acute mesenteric infarction with thrombosis**
    1. Acute mesenteric ischemia secondary to thrombosis is treated initially with a papaverine infusion started at angiography. Patients without peritoneal signs with minor thrombi may be treated with papaverine only.
    2. Patients with major thrombi with good collateral vasculature, without peritoneal signs, may be observed in the hospital without a papaverine infusion. Patients with peritoneal signs and documented thrombosis require laparotomy.

References: See page 113.

Intestinal Obstruction

I. Clinical evaluation
- **A.** Intestinal obstruction is characterized by nausea, vomiting, cramps, and obstipation. Suspected intestinal obstruction requires immediate surgical consultation.

Intestinal Obstruction

- **B. Small-bowel obstruction.** Auscultation may reveal high-pitched rushes or tinkles that coincide with episodes of cramping. Pain usually is epigastric or periumbilical.
    1. **Proximal obstruction.** Frequent non-bilious vomiting is prominent if the obstruction is proximal to the ampulla of Vater. Colicky pain occurs at frequent intervals (2-5 minutes). Obstipation may not occur until late, and distention is minimal or absent.
    2. **Distal obstruction.** Vomiting is bilious and less frequent. The vomiting may be feculent if the obstruction has been long-standing. Colicky pain occurs at intervals of 10 minutes or more, and it is less intense. A dull ache may persist between cramps. Distention increases gradually.
- **C. Colonic obstruction**
    1. Colonic obstruction is caused by colon cancer in 60-70% of cases, and diverticulitis and volvulus account for 30%. Obstruction is more common in the left colon than the right.
    2. Milder attacks of pain often occur in the weeks preceding the acute episode. Colic is perceived in the lower abdomen or suprapubically, and obstipation and distention are characteristic. Nausea is common, and vomiting may occur.
    3. Tenderness is usually mild in uncomplicated colonic obstruction. Rectal exam or sigmoidoscopy may detect an obstructing lesion.
- **D. Colonic pseudo-obstruction (Ogilvie's syndrome)** may occur in the elderly, bedridden or institutionalized individual, often after recent surgery.
- **E. Strangulated obstruction** is characterized by constant pain, fever, tachycardia, peritoneal signs, a tender abdominal mass, and leukocytosis.
- **F. Laboratory evaluation of intestinal obstruction**
    1. **Hypokalemic alkalosis** is the most common metabolic abnormality resulting from vomiting and fluid loss. Elevated BUN and creatinine suggests significant hypovolemia. Hypochloremic acidosis with increased anion gap may occur with strangulated obstruction.
    2. **Leukocyte count** frequently is normal in uncomplicated obstruction; however, leukocytosis suggests strangulation.
    3. **Serum amylase** may be elevated with bowel infarction.
- **G. Radiography**
    1. **Plain films**
        a. **Small-bowel obstruction.** Plain radiographs may demonstrate multiple air-fluid levels with dilated loops of small intestine, but no colonic gas. Proximal jejunal obstruction may not cause dilatation. Distal obstruction is characterized by a ladder pattern of dilated loops of bowel.
        b. **Colonic obstruction.** Obstructive lesions usually are located in the left colon and rectum and cause distention of the proximal colon. Dilated colon has a peripheral location within the abdomen, and haustral markings are present and valvulae conniventes are absent.
    2. **Contrast studies**
        a. **Barium contrast enema.** In colonic obstruction, a single-column contrast study with a water-soluble contrast enema should be performed. Contrast enema is contraindicated in obstruction from acute diverticulitis or in the presence of toxic megacolon.
        b. **Upper GI series.** In acute small bowel obstruction, plain films are usually sufficient. An upper GI series may be useful in partial small bowel obstruction.

H. Endoscopy
1. **Upper endoscopy** is the best test in obstruction of the gastric outlet or duodenum.
2. **Colonoscopy** can confirm the diagnosis of colon obstruction by cancer. Non-strangulated volvulus can often be reduced endoscopically, and elective resection can be completed at a later time.

References: See page 113.

Acute Pancreatitis

The incidence of acute pancreatitis ranges from 54 to 238 episodes per 1 million per year. Patients with mild pancreatitis respond well to conservative therapy, but those with severe pancreatitis may have a progressively downhill course to respiratory failure, sepsis, and death (less than 10%).

I. Etiology
A. **Alcohol-induced pancreatitis.** Consumption of large quantities of alcohol may cause acute pancreatitis.
B. **Cholelithiasis.** Common bile duct or pancreatic duct obstruction by a stone may cause acute pancreatitis. (90% of all cases of pancreatitis occur secondary to alcohol consumption or cholelithiasis).
C. **Idiopathic pancreatitis.** The cause of pancreatitis cannot be determined in 10 percent of patients.
D. **Hypertriglyceridemia.** Elevation of serum triglycerides (>l,000mg/dL) has been linked with acute pancreatitis.
E. **Pancreatic duct disruption.** In younger patients, a malformation of the pancreatic ducts (eg, pancreatic divisum) with subsequent obstruction is often the cause of pancreatitis. In older patients without an apparent underlying etiology, cancerous lesions of the ampulla of Vater, pancreas or duodenum must be ruled out as possible causes of obstructive pancreatitis.
F. **Iatrogenic pancreatitis.** Radiocontrast studies of the hepatobiliary system (eg, cholangiogram, ERCP) can cause acute pancreatitis in 2-3% of patients undergoing studies.
G. **Trauma.** Blunt or penetrating trauma of any kind to the peri-pancreatic or peri-hepatic regions may induce acute pancreatitis. Extensive surgical manipulation can also induce pancreatitis during laparotomy.

Causes of Acute Pancreatitis	
Alcoholism	Infections
Cholelithiasis	Microlithiasis
Drugs	Pancreas divisum
Hypertriglyceridemia	Trauma
Idiopathic causes	

84 Acute Pancreatitis

Medications Associated with Acute Pancreatitis	
Definitive Association: Azathioprine (Imuran) Sulfonamides Thiazide diuretics Furosemide (Lasix) Estrogens Tetracyclines Valproic acid (Depakote) Pentamidine Didanosine (Videx)	**Probable Association:** Acetaminophen Nitrofurantoin Methyldopa Erythromycin Salicylates Metronidazole NSAIDS ACE-inhibitors

II. **Pathophysiology.** Acute pancreatitis results when an initiating event causes the extrusion of zymogen granules, from pancreatic acinar cells, into the interstitium of the pancreas. Zymogen particles cause the activation of trypsinogen into trypsin. Trypsin causes auto-digestion of pancreatic tissues.

III. **Clinical presentation**
   A. **Signs and symptoms.** Pancreatitis usually presents with mid-epigastric pain that radiates to the back, associated with nausea and vomiting. The pain is sudden in onset, progressively increases in intensity, and becomes constant. The severity of pain often causes the patient to move continuously in search of a more comfortable position.
   B. **Physical examination**
      1. Patients with acute pancreatitis often appear very ill. Findings that suggest severe pancreatitis include hypotension and tachypnea with decreased basilar breath sounds. Flank ecchymoses (Grey Tuner's Sign) or periumbilical ecchymoses (Cullen's sign) may be indicative of hemorrhagic pancreatitis.
      2. Abdominal distension and tenderness in the epigastrium are common. Fever and tachycardia are often present. Guarding, rebound tenderness, and hypoactive or absent bowel sounds indicate peritoneal irritation. Deep palpation of abdominal organs should be avoided in the setting of suspected pancreatitis.

IV. **Laboratory testing**
   A. **Leukocytosis.** An elevated WBC with a left shift and elevated hematocrit (indicating hemoconcentration) and hyperglycemia are common. Pre-renal azotemia may result from dehydration. Hypoalbuminemia, hypertriglyceridemia, hypocalcemia, hyperbilirubinemia, and mild elevations of transaminases and alkaline phosphatase are common.
   B. **Elevated amylase.** An elevated amylase level often confirms the clinical diagnosis of pancreatitis.
   C. **Elevated lipase.** Lipase measurements are more specific for pancreatitis than amylase levels, but less sensitive. Hyperlipasemia may also occur in patients with renal failure, perforated ulcer disease, bowel infarction and bowel obstruction.
   D. **Abdominal Radiographs** may reveal non-specific findings of pancreatitis, such as "sentinel loops" (dilated loops of small bowel in the vicinity of the pancreas), ileus and, pancreatic calcifications.
   E. **Ultrasonography** demonstrates the entire pancreas in only 20 percent of patients with acute pancreatitis. Its greatest utility is in evaluation of patients with possible gallstone disease.
   F. **Helical high resolution computed tomography** is the imaging modality of choice in acute pancreatitis. CT findings will be normal in 14-29% of

patients with mild pancreatitis. Pancreatic necrosis, pseudocysts and abscesses are readily detected by CT.

Selected Conditions Other Than Pancreatitis Associated with Amylase Elevation

Carcinoma of the pancreas	Acute alcoholism
Common bile duct obstruction	Diabetic ketoacidosis
Post-ERCP	Lung cancer
Mesenteric infarction	Ovarian neoplasm
Pancreatic trauma	Renal failure
Perforated viscus	Ruptured ectopic pregnancy
Renal failure	Salivary gland infection
	Macroamylasemia

V. Prognosis. Ranson's criteria is used to determine prognosis in acute pancreatitis. Patients with two or fewer risk factors have a mortality rate of less than 1 percent, those with three or four risk-factors a mortality rate of 16 percent, five or six risk factors, a mortality rate of 40 percent, and seven or eight risk factors, a mortality rate approaching 100 percent.

Ranson's Criteria for Acute Pancreatitis

At admission	During initial 48 hours
1. Age >55 years 2. WBC >16,000/mm^3 3. Blood glucose >200 mg/dL 4. Serum LDH >350 IU/L 5. AST >250 U/L	1. Hematocrit drop >10% 2. BUN rise >5 mg/dL 3. Arterial pO$_2$ <60 mm Hg 4. Base deficit >4 mEq/L 5. Serum calcium <8.0 mg/dL 6. Estimated fluid sequestration >6 L

VI. Treatment of pancreatitis

A. Expectant management. Most cases of acute pancreatitis will improve within three to seven days. Management consists of prevention of complications of severe pancreatitis.

B. NPO and bowel rest. Patients should take nothing by mouth. Total parenteral nutrition should be instituted for those patients fasting for more than five days. A nasogastric tube is warranted if vomiting or ileus.

C. IV fluid resuscitation. Vigorous intravenous hydration is necessary. A decrease in urine output to less than 30 mL per hour is an indication of inadequate fluid replacement.

D. Pain control. Morphine is discouraged because it may cause Oddi's sphincter spasm, which may exacerbate the pancreatitis. Meperidine (Demerol), 25-100 mg IV/IM q4-6h, is favored. Ketorolac (Toradol), 60 mg IM/IV, then 15-30 mg IM/IV q6h, is also used.

E. Antibiotics. Routine use of antibiotics is not recommended in most cases of acute pancreatitis. In cases of infectious pancreatitis, treatment with cefoxitin (1-2 g IV q6h), cefotetan (1-2 g IV q12h), imipenem (1.0 gm IV q6h), or ampicillin/sulbactam (1.5-3.0 g IV q6h) may be appropriate.

F. Alcohol withdrawal prophylaxis. Alcoholics may require alcohol withdrawal prophylaxis with lorazepam (Ativan) 1-2mg IM/IV q4-6h as needed x 3 days, thiamine 100mg IM/IV qd x 3 days, folic acid 1 mg

IM/IV qd x 3 days, multivitamin qd.
- **G. Octreotide.** Somatostatin is also a potent inhibitor of pancreatic exocrine secretion. Octreotide is a somatostatin analogue, which has been effective in reducing mortality from bile-induced pancreatitis. Clinical trials, however, have failed to document a significant reduction in mortality
- **H. Blood sugar monitoring and insulin administration.** Serum glucose levels should be monitored.

VII. Complications
- A. Chronic pancreatitis
- B. Severe hemorrhagic pancreatitis
- C. Pancreatic pseudocysts
- D. Infectious pancreatitis with development of sepsis (occurs in up to 5% of all patients with pancreatitis)
- E. Portal vein thrombosis

References: See page 113.

Acute Cholecystitis

Russell A. Williams, MD

Acute cholecystitis is a bacterial inflammation of the gallbladder which may cause severe peritonitis. Gallstones are present in the gallbladder in about 95% of cases. The incidence of acute calculous cholecystitis is higher in females, with a female-to-male ratio of 3:1 up to the age of 50 and a ratio of 1.5:1 thereafter.

I. Pathophysiology.
Patients who have symptoms from gallstones have an elective cholecystectomy to avoid acute cholecystitis and its complications. Acute calculous cholecystitis is caused by obstruction of the cystic duct by a stone. Positive bacterial cultures of bile or gallbladder wall are found in 50% to 75% of cases.

II. Clinical evaluation
- **A.** Persistent pain in the area of the gallbladder is present in almost every case. Frequently, the pain develops after ingestion of a meal. The pain is usually in the right upper quadrant, the epigastrium, or both.
- **B.** The pain often radiates toward the tip of the scapula. Pain in the right shoulder is present when the diaphragm is irritated by the inflammation.
- **C.** Nausea and vomiting occur in 60% to 70% of patients.

III. Physical examination
- **A.** Fever is present in about 80% of patients. The most common and reliable finding on physical examination is tenderness in the right upper quadrant, the epigastrium, or both. About half of all patients have muscle rigidity in the right upper quadrant, and about one fourth have rebound tenderness.
- **B.** Murphy's sign, consisting of inspiratory arrest during deep palpation of the right upper quadrant, is not a consistent finding but is almost pathognomonic when present. A mass in the region of the gallbladder is palpable in about 40%.

IV. Laboratory evaluation and imaging studies
- **A. White blood cell count** is elevated in 85% of cases. One half have elevation of the serum bilirubin, and the serum amylase is increased in one third.

- **B. Radionuclide scan (HIDA scan).** The specific test for acute cholecystitis is the HIDA scan. Normally, the scan outlines the liver and the extrahepatic biliary tract, including the gallbladder, and shows the nuclide flowing into the upper small intestine. In acute cholecystitis, the gallbladder is not seen on the scan. Radionuclide has a sensitivity of almost 100% and a specificity of 95%.
- **C. Ultrasound.** Calculi within the gallbladder can be accurately detected by ultrasonography, but this test is not specific for acute calculous cholecystitis. A thickened gallbladder wall and pericholecystic fluid are sometimes present.

V. Differential diagnosis. Acute appendicitis, perforated or penetrating duodenal ulcer, acute or perforated gastric ulcer, and acute pancreatitis. In approximately 15% of cases of acute cholecystitis, the serum amylase is elevated, suggesting the possibility of acute pancreatitis.

VI. Treatment
- **A.** Patients suspected of having acute cholecystitis should be hospitalized. Intravenous crystalloids should be given to restore intravascular volume. Preoperative management should include administration of an antibiotic that is effective against gram-positive and -negative aerobes and anaerobes. Those present most frequently are *Escherichia coli*, *Klebsiella* species, *Streptococcus faecalis*, *Clostridium welchii*, *Proteus* species, *Enterobacter* species, and anaerobic *Streptococcus* species.
- **B.** A second-generation cephalosporin is recommended for most cases of acute cholecystitis and reservation of the triple drug combination for patients who are seriously ill with sepsis. Antibiotic therapy should be initiated as soon as the diagnosis is made and should be continued for 24 hours postoperatively, unless peritonitis is severe, in which case it should continue for 7 days.
  1. Ampicillin 1-3.0 gm IV q6h **OR**
  2. Ampicillin-sulbactam (Unasyn) 1.5-3.0 gm IV q6h **AND**
  3. Gentamicin, 1.5-2 mg/kg, then 2-5 mg/kg/d IV.
  4. Cefoxitin (Mefoxin) 1-2 gm IV q6-8h.
  5. Ticarcillin/clavulanate (Timentin) 3.1 g IV q4-6h.
  6. Piperacillin/tazobactam (Zosyn) 4.5 gm IV q6h.
  7. Meperidine (Demerol) 50-100 mg IV/IM q4-6h prn pain.
- **C.** The definitive treatment of acute cholecystitis is early laparoscopic cholecystectomy. Operative cholangiography is routinely performed unless the extent of inflammation makes it unsafe.

Laparoscopic Cholecystectomy Procedure

I. Advantages of laparoscopic surgery: Usually less postoperative pain, reduced recovery time; several small puncture wounds instead of a large surgical incision, and early return to work.

II. Contraindications to laparoscopic cholecystectomy: Adhesions, extreme gallbladder scarring, severe acute inflammation, and bleeding.

III. Technique
- **A.** Preoperative antibiotic therapy with cefoxitin (Mefoxin) 1-2 gm IV q6h is usually used routinely. The procedure is performed with the patient under general or epidural anesthesia.
- **B.** The stomach is decompressed with a nasogastric tube to facilitate exposure. With the patient in the supine position, a 2-cm incision is made

Laparoscopic Cholecystectomy Procedure

superior or inferior to the umbilicus. Using S-shaped retractors, the fascia is identified and grasped with a small Kocher or Allis clamp. The fascia is elevated and incised to allow for easy admission of a finger to confirm entrance into the abdominal cavity and sweep away any adhesions. A U-stitch is placed using an absorbable suture. The Hasson cannula is inserted and secured with the suture used for the U-stitch.

C. After setting the insufflator to an insufflation pressure of 12 mm Hg, CO_2 is instilled at a low flow (1 L/min) into the abdominal cavity through the Hasson cannula. Approximately 1 L CO_2 is instilled at a low flow rate, and then the flow rate is adjusted to the maximum (20 L/min). The endoscope is inserted, and the abdominal and pelvic cavities are inspected.

D. The patient is placed in reverse Trendelenburg position to allow the colon and omentum to fall inferiorly. After the pelvis and upper abdomen are visually inspected, a 10-mm cannula is inserted two thirds of the way between the umbilicus and the xiphisternum just to the right of the midline. A 5-mm cannula is inserted 3 cm inferior to the costal margin in the midclavicular line, and a second 5-mm cannula is inserted 4 cm inferior to the costal margin in the midaxillary line. All three cannulas are inserted using a trocar under direct endoscopic vision. The umbilical cannula is used for the endoscope and CO2 inflow, and the epigastric port is used for dissection. Through the most lateral right subcostal cannula, a grasper retracts the dome of the gallbladder over the liver toward the right diaphragm. Through the other subcostal cannula, a grasper retracts the neck of the gallbladder laterally and anteriorly.

E. Adhesions are dissected off of the gallbladder, and dissection is begun at the neck of the gallbladder and proceeds along the cystic duct. After the cystic duct and artery have been identified by removal of the peritoneum overlying these structures, a titanium clip is placed at the junction of the neck and cystic duct. A cholangiogram is performed by partially transecting the cystic duct using scissors. The cholangiocatheter is inserted into the cholecystodochotomy, and a cholangiogram is performed using 30% Renografin.

F. If the cholangiogram is normal, the catheter is removed and the cystic duct is secured just inferior to the ductotomy with two titanium clips and divided. The cystic artery is clipped and divided. The infundibulum and neck of the gallbladder are rotated medially or laterally, and the peritoneal reflection onto the gallbladder is incised using the hook cautery. The gallbladder is dissected from its bed, and before the last attachments at the dome are divided, the gallbladder bed is irrigated and inspected for bleeding and bile leaks. The stumps of the cystic duct and artery are inspected for bleeding and bile leaks.

G. When hemostasis is attained, the remaining attachments between the gallbladder and the liver are divided and the gallbladder is positioned just superior to the liver. The laparoscope and CO_2 insufflation tubing are transferred to the epigastric cannula, and the extraction sack is passed under direct visualization through the umbilical cannula. The sack is opened, and the gallbladder placed in the bag and extracted.

H. The umbilical incision is closed under direct visualization by tying the U-stitch. The subcostal cannulas are removed under direct visualization. The epigastric cannula is positioned over the liver away from the omentum, CO_2 insufflation stopped, and residual CO_2 allowed to escape from the abdomen through the cannula. The cannula is removed, and the incisions are closed with a subcuticular stitch and sterile strips. Dressings are placed over the incisions, and the nasogastric tube and Foley catheter are removed. The patient may be discharged after observation. Most patients can be discharged within a few hours.

Open Cholecystectomy Procedure

A. After induction of anesthesia place a nasogastric tube to decompress the stomach. The most commonly used incision is Kocher's right subcostal. Place incision 4 cm below and parallel to the costal margin, and extend it from the midline to the anterior axillary line. Open the anterior rectus sheath with a knife in the line of the incision. Divide the rectus muscle with cautery, and open the peritoneum between forceps.

B. Systematically explore the peritoneal cavity and note the appearance of the hiatus, stomach, duodenum, liver, pancreas, intestines, and kidneys. Palpate the gallbladder from the ampulla towards the fundus, then palpate the common duct, noting any dilation or foreign bodies. Carefully palpate the colon for neoplasms.

C. Grasp the gallbladder with a Rochester-Pean clamp near the fundus. Hold forceps in one hand, and introduce the right hand over the right lobe of the liver, permitting the liver to descend. Divide any adhesions to the omentum, colon or duodenum, and place a pack over these structures. Retract the structures inferiorly with a broad-bladed Deaver's retractor.

D. Inspect the anatomy of the biliary tree by carefully dividing the peritoneum covering the anterior aspect of the cystic duct, and continue dissecting into the anterior layer of the lesser omentum overlying the common bile duct. Bluntly dissect with a dissector (Kitner), exposing Charcot's triangle bounded by the cystic duct, common bile duct and inferior border of the liver. The cystic artery should be seen in this triangle. Carefully observe the arrangement of the duct system and arterial supply. Do not divide any structure until the anatomy has been identified, including the cystic duct and common bile duct.

E. Pass a ligature around the cystic duct with a right-angle clamp, and make a loose knot near the common duct. Partially divide the cystic duct below the infundibulum, and place a small polyethylene catheter attached to a syringe filled with saline into the cystic duct for 1-2 cm. Tighten the ligature holding the catheter in position.

F. Attach a second syringe containing contrast material to the catheter, and remove all instruments. Place a sterile sheet, and slowly inject 10-15 cc of diluted dye into the common duct. An operative cholangiogram should be performed to detect stones and evaluate the duct system.

G. Palpate the lower end of common bile duct, pancreas, and the foramen of Winslow. Palpate the ampulla, checking for stones or tumor. Hold the forceps on the gallbladder in the left hand, and clear the cystic artery of soft tissue with a pledget held in forceps. Follow the artery to the gallbladder, and clamp it with a right angle clamp. Divide and ligate the artery close to the edge of the gallbladder, using clips or 000 silk.

H. Reaffirm the junction of the cystic duct with the common bile, then completely divide the exposed cystic duct, leaving a stump of 5 mm.

I. Incise the peritoneum anteriorly over the gallbladder with a scalpel. Elevate the peritoneum from the gallbladder, and separate the gallbladder gently with sharp and blunt dissection. Tissue strands containing vessels should be cauterized before division.

J. Inspect the gallbladder bed for bleeding and cauterize and/or ligate any bleeding areas. Control any persistent oozing from the bed with a small pack of hemostatic gauze.

K. Irrigate the site with saline. If there is excessive fluid present, place a soft rubber Penrose drain or closed suction drain in the area of the dissection, and bring it out through a separate stab wound in the right upper quadrant. Inspect the operative field, including the ligatures on the arteries and the cystic duct. Approximate the peritoneum with continuous nonabsorbable suture.

L. Irrigate the wound with saline and approximate the rectus fascia and fascia of the oblique muscles with interrupted, nonabsorbable sutures. Irrigate the subcutaneous space with saline, and close the skin with staples, or absorbable subcuticular sutures.

Choledocholithiasis

Choledocholithiasis results when gallstones pass from the gallbladder through the cystic duct into the common duct.

I. **Clinical evaluation**
   A. Patients with choledocholithiasis generally present with jaundice. The patient may have pain or symptoms from associated biliary colic or acute cholecystitis.
   B. **Physical examination.** Icterus is typical unless there is associated acute cholecystitis. Ultrasonography can demonstrate gallstones in the gallbladder and in the common bile duct in 20-50% of patients with choledocholithiasis.
   C. The diagnosis depends on demonstrating enlarged common bile and intrahepatic ducts associated with abnormal liver function tests.
   D. **Alkaline phosphatase and bilirubin** are usually elevated.
   E. **Ultrasound** may reveal a dilated common bile duct, and stones may be seen. Frequently, gallstones in the lower common bile duct cannot be demonstrated by ultrasonography because of overlying bowel gas.
   F. **Endoscopic retrograde cholangiopancreatography (ERCP) or percutaneous transhepatic cholangiography (PTC)** are often used to confirm the diagnosis. Theses tests can opacify the biliary tree and demonstrate intraductal stones.

II. **Management of choledocholithiasis**
   A. All jaundiced patients and those known to have many, large, or intrahepatic stones should have preoperative ERCP to rule out malignancy and retrieve the stones.
   B. Preoperative ERCP with sphincterotomy should be performed in all patients who are at high risk of common bile duct stones or in whom common bile duct stones have been demonstrated. Laparoscopic cholecystectomy may be completed later.
   C. If ERCP is unsuccessful at clearing the common bile duct, the patient may require a laparoscopic or open cholecystectomy.

Disorders of the Breast

John A. Butler, MD

Breast Cancer Screening and Diagnosis

Breast cancer is the second most commonly diagnosed cancer among women, after skin cancer. Approximately 182,800 new cases of invasive breast cancer are diagnosed in the United States per year. The incidence of breast cancer increases with age. White women are more likely to develop breast cancer than black women. The incidence of breast cancer in white women is about 113 cases per 100,000 women and in black women, 100 cases per 100,000.

I. Risk factors

Risk Factors for Breast Cancer	
Age greater than 50 years Prior history of breast cancer Family history Early menarche, before age 12 Late menopause, after age 50 Nulliparity	Age greater than 30 at first birth Obesity High socioeconomic status Atypical hyperplasia on biopsy Ionizing radiation exposure

- **A.** Family history is highly significant in a first-degree relative (ie, mother, sister, daughter), especially if the cancer has been diagnosed premenopausally. Women who have premenopausal first-degree relatives with breast cancer have a three- to fourfold increased risk of breast cancer. Having several second-degree relatives with breast cancer may further increase the risk of breast cancer. Most women with breast cancer have no identifiable risk factors.
- **B.** Approximately 8 percent of all cases of breast cancer are hereditary. About one-half of these cases are attributed to mutations in the BRCA1 and BRCA2 genes. Hereditary breast cancer commonly occurs in premenopausal women. Screening tests are available that detect BRCA mutations.

II. Diagnosis and evaluation

- **A. Clinical evaluation of a breast mass** should assess duration of the lesion, associated pain, relationship to the menstrual cycle or exogenous hormone use, and change in size since discovery. The presence of nipple discharge and its character (bloody or tea-colored, unilateral or bilateral, spontaneous or expressed) should be assessed.
- **B. Menstrual history.** The date of last menstrual period, age of menarche, age of menopause or surgical removal of the ovaries, previous pregnancies should be determined.
- **C. History of previous breast biopsies**, cyst aspiration, dates and results of previous mammograms should be determined.
- **D. Family history** should document breast cancer in relatives and the age at which family members were diagnosed.

III. Physical examination
A. The breasts should be inspected for asymmetry, deformity, skin retraction, erythema, peau d'orange (breast edema), and nipple retraction, discoloration, or inversion.
B. **Palpation**
 1. The breasts should be palpated while the patient is sitting and then supine with the ipsilateral arm extended. The entire breast should be palpated systematically. The mass should be evaluated for size, shape, texture, tenderness, fixation to skin or chest wall.
 2. A mass that is suspicious for breast cancer is usually solitary, discrete and hard. In some instances, it is fixed to the skin or the muscle. A suspicious mass is usually unilateral and nontender. Sometimes, an area of thickening may represent cancer. Breast cancer is rarely bilateral. The nipples should be expressed for discharge.
 3. The axillae should be palpated for adenopathy, with an assessment of size of the lymph nodes, number, and fixation.

IV. Mammography.
Screening mammograms are recommended every year for asymptomatic women 40 years and older. Unfortunately, only 60 percent of cancers are diagnosed at a local stage.

Screening for Breast Cancer in Women	
Age	American Cancer Society guidelines
20 to 39 years	Clinical breast examination every three years Monthly self-examination of breasts
Age 40 years and older	Annual mammogram Annual clinical breast examination Monthly self-examination of breasts

V. Methods of breast biopsy
A. **Palpable masses.** Fine-needle aspiration biopsy (**FNAB**) has a sensitivity ranging from 90-98%. Nondiagnostic aspirates require surgical biopsy.
 1. The skin is prepped with alcohol and the lesion is immobilized with the nonoperating hand. A 10 mL syringe, with a 14 gauge needle, is introduced in to the central portion of the mass at a 90° angle. When the needle enters the mass, suction is applied by retracting the plunger, and the needle is advanced. The needle is directed into different areas of the mass while maintaining suction on the syringe.
 2. Suction is slowly released before the needle is withdrawn from the mass. The contents of the needle are placed onto glass slides for pathologic examination.
 3. Excisional biopsy is done when needle biopsies are negative but the mass is clinically suspected of malignancy.
B. **Stereotactic core needle biopsy.** Using a computer-driven stereotactic unit, the lesion is localized in three dimensions, and an automated biopsy needle obtains samples. The sensitivity and specificity of this technique are 95-100% and 94-98%, respectively.

C. Nonpalpable lesions
1. Needle localized biopsy
   a. Under mammographic guidance, a needle and hookwire are placed into the breast parenchyma adjacent to the lesion. The patient is taken to the operating room along with mammograms for an excisional breast biopsy.
   b. The skin and underlying tissues are infiltrated with 1% lidocaine with epinephrine. For lesions located within 5 cm of the nipple, a periareolar incision may be used or use a curved incision located over the mass and parallel to the areola. Incise the skin and subcutaneous fat, then palpate the lesion and excise the mass.
   c. After removal of the specimen, a specimen x-ray is performed to confirm that the lesion has been removed. The specimen can then be sent fresh for pathologic analysis.
   d. Close the subcutaneous tissues with a 4-0 chromic catgut suture, and close the skin with 4-0 subcuticular suture.
D. Ultrasonography.
Screening is useful to differentiate between solid and cystic breast masses when a palpable mass is not well seen on a mammogram. Ultrasonography is especially helpful in young women with dense breast tissue when a palpable mass is not visualized on a mammogram. Ultrasonography is not used for routine screening because microcalcifications are not visualized and the yield of carcinomas is negligible.

References: See page 113.

Breast Cysts

I. Clinical evaluation
   A. A breast cyst is palpable as a smooth, mobile, well-defined mass. If the cyst is tense, the texture may be very firm, resembling a cancer. Aspiration will determine whether the lesion is solid or cystic. Breast cyst fluid may vary from straw-colored to dark green. Cytology is not routinely necessary. The cyst should be aspirated completely.
   B. If a mass remains after drainage or if the fluid is bloody, excisional biopsy is indicated. If no palpable mass is felt after drainage, the patient should be reexamined in 3-4 weeks to determine whether the cyst recurs. Recurrent cysts can be re-aspirated. Repeated recurrence of the cyst requires an open biopsy to exclude intracystic tumor.
   C. **Nonpalpable cysts.** If the cyst wall is seen clearly on ultrasound and there is no interior debris or intracystic tumor, these simple cysts do not need to be aspirated. Any irregularity of the cyst wall or debris within the cyst requires a needle localized biopsy.

Fibroadenomas

I. Clinical evaluation
A. Fibroadenomas frequently present in young women as firm, smooth, lobulated masses that are highly mobile. They have a benign appearance on mammography and are solid by ultrasound.
B. A tissue diagnosis can be obtained by fine needle aspiration biopsy or excisional biopsy.

II. Management of fibroadenomas
A. Fibroadenomas may be followed conservatively after the diagnosis has been made. If the mass grows, it should be excised.
B. Large fibroadenomas (>2.5 cm) should usually be excised. Often fibroadenomas will grow in the presence of hormonal stimulation, such as pregnancy.

References: See page 113.

Breast Cancer

The initial management of the breast cancer patient consists of assigning a clinical stage based on examination. The stage may be altered once the final pathology of the tumor has been determined. Staging of breast cancer is based on the TNM staging system.

I. **Preoperative staging in stage I and II breast cancer.** Preoperative workup should include a CBC, SMA18, and chest x-ray. If elevated alkaline phosphatase or hypercalcemia is present, a bone scan should be completed. Abnormal liver function tests should be investigated with a CT scan of the liver.

American Joint Committee on Cancer TNM staging for breast cancer	
Stage	**Description**
Tumor	
TX	Primary tumor not assessable
T0	No evidence of primary tumor
Tis	Carcinoma in situ
T1	Tumor ≤2 cm in greatest dimension
T1a	Tumor ≤0.5 cm in greatest dimension
T1b	Tumor >0.5 cm but not > 1 cm
T1c	Tumor >1 cm but not >2 cm
T2	Tumor >2 cm but <5 cm in greatest dimension
T3	Tumor >5 cm in greatest dimension
T4	Tumor of any size with direct extension into the chest wall or skin
T4a	Extension to chest wall (ribs, intercostal muscles, or serratus anterior)
T4b	Peau d'orange, ulceration, or satellite skin nodules
T4c	T4a plus b
T4d	Inflammatory breast cancer

Stage	Description
Regional lymph nodes	
NX	Regional lymph nodes not assessable
N0	No regional lymph node involvement
N1	Metastasis to movable ipsilateral axillary lymph nodes
N2	Metastases to ipsilateral axillary lymph nodes fixed to one another or to other structures
N3	Metastases to ipsilateral internal mammary lymph nodes
Distant metastases	
MX	Non-accessible presence of distant metastases
M0	No distant metastases
M1	Existent distant metastases (including ipsilateral supraclavicular nodes)

American Joint Committee on Cancer classification for breast cancer based on TNM criteria

Stage	Tumor	Nodes	Metastases
0	Tis	N0	M0
I	T1	N0	M0
IIA	T0, 1 T2	N1 N0	M0 M0
IIB	T2 T3	N1 N0	M0 M0
IIIA	T0, 1, 2 T3	N2 N1, 2	M0 M0
IIIB	T4 Any T	Any N N3	M0 M0
IV	Any T	Any N	M1

II. Surgical options for stage I and II breast cancer

A. Breast conservation therapy (BCT) has been shown to result in survival and local recurrence rates equivalent to modified radical mastectomy; therefore, breast conservation is the preferred therapy for stage I and II breast cancer. The technique includes lumpectomy, axillary lymph node dissection, and breast irradiation.

1. Contraindications to BCT
   a. Contraindications to radiotherapy (ie, prior breast irradiation, ongoing pregnancy)
   b. Steroid-dependent collagen vascular disease
   c. Tumor-breast ratio that would result in an unacceptable cosmetic result (eg, a large tumor in a small breast)
   d. Diffuse, malignant microcalcifications on mammography

e. Tumor greater than 5 cm in diameter
  2. **Lumpectomy technique.** Incisions should be curvilinear and parallel with the nipple. A gross margin of 1 cm should be removed. The lumpectomy specimen is given immediately to the pathologist for inking and for an assessment of the gross margins. Subcutaneous tissue is closed, and the skin is approximated with a subcuticular suture.
  3. Follow-up following BCT consists of a physical examination every 3-4 months for the first 3 years, every 6 months for the next 2-3 years, then yearly. A SMA18 and CBC are done at each visit and a chest x-ray is done yearly.
  4. A posttreatment mammography of the treated side is done 6 months after the completion of radiotherapy, then every 6 months for the first 2 years, followed by annual mammograms. Yearly mammography should be performed on the opposite breast.
 B. **Modified radical mastectomy** consists of a total mastectomy and an axillary node dissection. In staging axillary lymphadenectomy, levels I and II are removed routinely. Reconstruction of the breast should be offered to all patients undergoing mastectomy. Physical examination schedule and blood work are the same as for lumpectomy. The chest wall should be examined for of recurrence. Mammography of the opposite breast should continue yearly.
III. **Locally advanced breast cancer (LABC)** consists of T3 N0 (stage IIB), IIIA, and IIIB breast cancer. All LABC patients should undergo staging with CBC, SMA18, bone scan, and CT scan of chest and abdomen.
 A. **Noninflammatory LABC.** Multimodality therapy consists of neoadjuvant chemotherapy (ie, given before surgery), modified radical mastectomy, radiotherapy to the chest wall, axilla and supraclavicular nodes, and further chemotherapy.
 B. **Inflammatory LABC (T4d).** Inflammatory breast cancer is characterized by erythema of the skin, skin edema, warmth, tenderness, and an underlying tumor mass. Treatment requires aggressive multi-modality therapy.
 C. **Follow-up.** Patients should be followed closely because they are at higher risk of local and distant recurrence.
IV. **Ductal carcinoma in situ (DCIS)** consist of Tis, stage 0 lesions. These lesions consists of malignant ductal cells that have not penetrated the basement membrane. DCIS is a precursor of invasive ductal cancer.
 A. **Physical examination** is usually normal with DCIS. The most common presentation is suspicious microcalcifications on mammography. DCIS can cause a nipple discharge or a palpable mass.
 B. **Surgical therapy**
  1. **BCT.** Lumpectomy and adjuvant radiotherapy are an alternative to mastectomy in well-localized DCIS when negative microscopic margins can be obtained.
  2. **Total mastectomy,** including removal of the nipple areolar complex and breast tissue, results in survival rates of 98-99%. An axillary dissection is not done routinely because the chance of nodal involvement is only 1-2%.

References: See page 113.

Urologic Disorders

C. Garo Gholdoian, MD
David A. Chamberlin, MD

Prostate Cancer

The average age at diagnosis of prostate cancer is 73 years. The prevalence of prostate cancer is 30% in men over the age of 50. One in six men will be diagnosed with prostate cancer during their lifetimes. Prostate cancer is the most common cancer in men except for skin cancer.

I. Clinical evaluation
- **A.** Prostate cancer is usually asymptomatic at presentation, and it is usually detected by abnormalities on rectal examination or a high serum prostate specific antigen (PSA) concentration.
- **B.** Prostate cancer can cause urinary urgency, nocturia, frequency, and hesitancy; these symptoms are more likely to be caused benign prostatic hypertrophy (BPH) than cancer. The new onset of erectile dysfunction raises the suspicion of prostate cancer.
- **C. Serum PSA elevation.** A total serum PSA concentration >4.0 ng/mL is considered abnormal, and is suspicious for prostate cancer. An elevated serum PSA between 4 to 10 ng/mL has a positive predictive value (PPV) of 21 percent, and a PSA above 10 ng/mL has a positive predictive value of 64 percent. Causes of an elevated PSA include benign prostatic hyperplasia, prostate cancer, prostatitis, and perineal trauma.
- **D. Abnormal prostate examination.** The PPV of an abnormal digital rectal examination for prostate cancer is 5 to 30 percent. All men with induration, asymmetry, or palpable nodularity of the prostate gland require further diagnostic studies to rule out prostate cancer. A serum PSA should be obtained prior to biopsy.

II. Screening for prostate cancer
- **A.** Age is the most important risk factor for prostate cancer. Prostate cancer rarely occurs before the age of 45, but the incidence rises rapidly thereafter. Prostate cancer is more common in black men.
- **B. Recommendations for screening.** The American Cancer Society recommends that serum prostate specific antigen testing and digital rectal examination should be offered annually to men 50 years of age and older who have a life expectancy of 10 years. Screening should begin at age 45 in patients at high-risk for prostate cancer (eg, African Americans and men with two or more first-degree relatives with prostate cancer). PSA testing is also recommended for men who ask their clinicians to make the decision about screening on their behalf. The American Urological Association also supports this policy.
- **C. If the serum PSA concentration is abnormal (>4.0 ng/mL),** the test should be repeated in four weeks for confirmation. The most common explanation for an elevated serum PSA value is BPH. A man who has a high serum PSA concentration should be treated with an antibiotic (trimethoprim-sulfamethoxazole ([Bactrim]) 1 DS tablet bid for 3 weeks) because prostatitis is a common cause of a high PSA. The PSA concentration should be repeated in 4 weeks. A return of the PSA to

normal is expected if prostatitis was solely responsible.

- **D. Prostate biopsy** is the gold standard for prostate cancer diagnosis. Transrectal biopsy is a simple office technique that requires no analgesia. In a standard ultrasound-guided biopsy, a specimen is removed with a biopsy gun from any suspicious areas (eg, by rectal examination or biopsy) followed by six to ten tissue cores from the base, midzone, and apical areas of the right and left lobes of the gland (sextant biopsies).

III. Diagnostic and staging evaluation of prostate cancer

A. The tumor-node-metastasis (TNM) system is the most popular method of staging prostate cancer. Men are usually assigned a clinical stage, or "c" stage, and a pathological stage, or "p" stage. The "c" stage is determined by the digital rectal examination, while the "p" stage is determined after a pathologist has evaluated a radical prostatectomy specimen.

IV. Staging of prostate cancer

Staging of Prostate Cancer by 2002 AJCC Staging System

Clinical tumor (cT) stage	Substage	
Stage cT1 Clinically inapparent tumor neither palpable nor visible by imaging	T1a	Tumor incidental histologic finding in five percent or less of tissue resected
	T1b	Tumor incidental histologic finding in more than five percent of tissue resected
	T1c	Tumor identified by needle biopsy (eg, because of elevated PSA)
Stage cT2 Tumor confined within the prostate	T2a	Tumor involves one-half of one lobe or less
	T2b	Tumor involves more than one-half of one lobe but not both lobes
	T2c	Tumor involving both lobes
Stage cT3	T3a	Extracapsular extension (Unilateral or bilateral)
	T3b	Tumor invades the seminal vesicle(s)
Stage cT4 Tumor is fixed or invades adjacent structures other than seminal vesicles: bladder neck, external sphincter, rectum, levator muscles, and/or pelvic wall.		

Prostate Cancer

Stage Grouping for Prostate Cancer, 2002 AJCC Criteria				
Stage I	T1a	N0	M0	G1*
Stage II	T1a	N0	M0	G2, 3-4
		N0	M0	Any G
		N0	M0	Any G
		N0	M0	Any G
		N0	M0	Any G
Stage III	T3	N0	M0	Any G
Stage IV	T4	N0	M0	Any G
	Any T	N1	M0	Any G
	Any T	Any N	M1	Any G

*Grade: tumor grade is assessed as follows:
Grade 1: Well differentiated (slight anaplasia), Gleason score 2-4
Grade 2: Moderately differentiated (moderate anaplasia) Gleason score 5-6
Grade 3-4: Poorly differentiated/undifferentiated (marked anaplasia) Gleason score 7-10

A. **Tumor histology (Gleason score).** Analysis of the tumor histology provides an index of prognosis and may guide local therapy. Gleason score of one represents the most well-differentiated appearance, and Gleason score ten represents the most poorly differentiated.

B. **Clinical staging**
  1. **Serum PSA.** This value is not used for staging, but may help to predict the local extent of disease in men with prostate cancer. There is a higher likelihood of finding organ-confined disease when the serum PSA concentration is less than 4.0 ng/mL. A serum PSA concentration of 4.1 to 10.0 ng/mL increases the likelihood of finding an organ-confined tumor larger than 0.5 mL, but also increases the odds of finding extracapsular extension by 5.1-fold. A serum PSA concentration higher than 10.0 ng/mL increases the likelihood of finding extraprostatic extension by 24 to 50-fold.
  2. **Radionuclide bone scan.** A positive radionuclide bone scan indicates extraprostatic spread and eliminates the potential for curative surgery. Bone scan need not be performed in a patient with clinical stage T1 or T2 cancer on physical examination, a Gleason score of six or less, and a serum PSA value less than 10 ng/mL.
  3. **CT scan** should be considered in men who are going to be treated with external beam radiation therapy, and in men who have a PSA >10 to 15 ng/mL or a Gleason score greater than six. These men have an increased likelihood of pelvic lymph node metastasis.
  4. **Endorectal coil magnetic resonance imaging (MRI)** of the prostate gland utilizing an endorectal probe can determine the likelihood of

either seminal vesicle involvement or extracapsular extension in patients who are thought to have clinically localized prostate cancer. The likelihood of cure with either radiation therapy or radical prostatectomy is low in these locally advanced patients, and surgery is usually not recommended.

V. Treatment for early prostate cancer (organ-confined)

A. The three standard therapies for men with early stage (organ-confined) prostate cancer are radical prostatectomy (RP), radiotherapy (RT), and watchful waiting. Hormone therapy is reserved for patients with locally advanced or metastatic prostate cancer.

B. **Radical prostatectomy**
  1. RP involves excising the entire prostate from the urethra and bladder, which are then reconnected. This treatment offers the best chance of long-term survival. The retropubic approach to RP permits pelvic lymph node sampling prior to prostate removal to confirm the presence or absence of metastases. The prostate is removed if the lymph nodes are free of disease.
  2. Fifteen-year progression-free survival rates have been reported to be 80 to 85 percent for men with organ-confined disease.
  3. **Complications**
     a. **Incontinence**. About 1.6 percent report no urinary control, 7 percent report frequent leakage, and 42 percent report occasional leakage.
     b. **Impotence**. The potency rate after surgery is 100 percent in men in their 40s, 55 percent for men in their 50s, 43 percent for men in their 60s, and 0 percent for men in their 70s.
  4. **Perineal prostatectomy** can be considered for men with lower grade and low volume tumors, such as those with Gleason score <6 and a serum PSA less than 10 ng/mL. The likelihood of extraprostatic disease is less than 5 percent in such patients, making pelvic lymph node dissection unnecessary.

C. **Radiation therapy**
  1. **Radiation therapy (RT)** does not require hospitalization and normal activity can usually be maintained during the course of treatment. Cure rates with RT appear to be comparable to those with RP for clinically localized disease for the first five years. Late recurrences following RT ten years or more after treatment occur more frequently than with RP.

D. **Watchful waiting**
  1. Watchful waiting describes patients who forego treatment. Such patients are followed with serum PSA measurements and digital rectal examination every three months for the first year, and then less frequently. Definitive or palliative therapy is initiated if a significant change in the serum PSA concentration or DRE occurs.
  2. Men with early stage disease (T0 to T2, NX, M0) were followed for ten years, and only 9 percent died of prostate cancer. The survival rate of this "watched" group was similar to the survival rate of the treated group.

E. **Recommendations**
  1. Early stage (organ-confined) prostate cancer is a curable disease in the majority of men. Surgery and radiation therapy offer equivalent survival outcomes for the first ten years after therapy; beyond that time, there is a higher risk of recurrence with radiation. Younger men

should undergo surgery because of the potential for late recurrence with radiation therapy. Older men may prefer radiation therapy.
2. Watchful waiting is not a good option for men with high-risk tumors (eg, Gleason score 7 or higher) unless they have significant comorbidity that suggests a markedly reduced life expectancy. The ideal candidate for watchful waiting is over the age of 70 to 75 with a life expectancy of 10 to 15 years or less who has a low grade tumor (eg, Gleason score 2 to 4).
F. **Endocrine therapy of advanced prostate carcinoma.** Treatment of stage IV prostate cancer involves surgical or medical castration. Total blockade with leuprolide (Lupron) plus flutamide (Eulexin) is slightly better than leuprolide alone. Orchiectomy is an outpatient procedure that is the safest and least expensive option. The incidence of impotence with orchiectomy is no different than with medical castration therapies.

References: See page 113.

Renal Colic

Approximately 5% of the U.S. population will pass a urinary tract stone during their lifetime.

I. Pathophysiology
  A. Calcium-containing stones are the most common (70%).
  B. Magnesium-ammonium-phosphate stones, also known as struvite stones, are almost always associated with urinary tract infection with urea-splitting bacteria, such as Proteus mirabilis.
  C. Uric acid stones are less common and are radiolucent, making diagnosis by plain films alone difficult.
  D. Cystine stones are rare and associated with cystinuria, a rare autosomal recessive hereditary disorder.

II. Clinical evaluation
  A. Renal colic is characterized as severe colicky pain that is intermittent and usually in the flank or lower abdomen. Patients usually cannot find a "comfortable position," and the pain often radiates to the testes or groin. A history of previous stones, poor fluid intake, urinary tract infections, or hematuria is common.
  B. Obstruction located at the ureteropelvic junction causes pure flank pain, while upper ureteral obstruction causes flank pain that radiates to the groin. Midureteral stones cause lower abdominal pain and may mimic appendicitis or diverticulitis, but without localized point tenderness or guarding. Lower ureteral stones may cause irritative voiding symptoms and scrotal or labial pain.
  C. Patients with nephrolithiasis generally complain of nausea and vomiting. They commonly have gross or microscopic hematuria, fever, and an increased white blood cell count may. Prior episodes of renal colic or a family history of renal stones is often reported.
  D. **Physical examination**
    1. Generally the patient is agitated, diaphoretic, and unable to find a comfortable position.
    2. Hypertension and tachycardia are common.
    3. Costovertebral angle tenderness is the classic physical finding; however, minimal abdominal tenderness without guarding, rebound or

rigidity may be present. Right or left lower quadrant tenderness or an enlarged kidney may sometimes be noted.

III. Differential diagnosis. Appendicitis, salpingitis, diverticulitis, pyelonephritis, ovarian torsion, prostatitis, ectopic pregnancy, bowel obstruction, carcinoma.

IV. Laboratory evaluation

   A. A urinalysis with microscopic, serum electrolytes, BUN, creatinine, complete blood count, and urine culture should be obtained. An elevated white blood cell count may be noted. A significant number of white cells in the urine also suggests infection.

   B. A plain abdominal film may demonstrate a calcification along the course of the urinary tract. Ninety percent of all calculi are radiopaque. Calcifications are frequently obscured by overlying bowel gas.

   C. Intravenous pyelogram. IVP is the gold standard for the diagnosis of urolithiasis, and it allows rapid assessment of the degree of obstruction, location of the stone and any renal function impairment. Acute ureteral obstruction may appear as a dense nephrogram with a delay in excretion of contrast.

   D. Ultrasound may be useful in patients with renal failure or an intravenous contrast allergy.

V. Management of renal calculi

   A. Most renal calculi will pass spontaneously, and only expectant management with hydration and analgesia is necessary. Obstruction associated with fever indicates urinary tract infection, and it requires prompt drainage with either a ureteral stent or percutaneous nephrostomy.

   B. Indications for admission
   1. High fever, uncontrollable pain
   2. Intractable nausea and vomiting with an inability to tolerate oral fluids
   3. Solitary kidney

   C. Inpatient management
   1. Vigorous intravenous hydration and intravenous antibiotics are important when infection is suspected. Parenteral narcotics are often necessary.
   2. Ketorolac (Toradol), 60 mg IM/IV, then 15-30 mg IM/IV q6h, is effective and provides a good alternative to narcotics.
   3. Strain all urine in an attempt to retrieve spontaneously passed stones for X-ray crystallographic analysis.
   4. Stones measuring 5 to 10 mm have a decreased likelihood of passage, and early elective intervention should be considered
   5. Extracorporeal shock-wave lithotripsy (ESWL) is the most common procedure for small renal or ureteral stones. Eighty percent of patients become stone-free after one treatment.
   6. Ureteroscopy with laser, ultrasound or electrohydraulic lithotripsy may be used as well. Open surgical stone removal is rarely necessary.

   D. Outpatient management
   1. Most patients with renal colic do not require admission. The majority of stones measuring less than 4 mm will pass spontaneously (90-95%), and 80% of these will pass within 4 weeks.
   2. Patients should increase intake of oral fluids, take narcotic pain medication, and strain all urine. Plain abdominal films may be used to assess movement of the stone.

   E. Follow-up care
   1. After the stone has passed, a metabolic evaluation is important

Urologic Emergencies

I. Acute urinary retention

A. Acute urinary retention is characterized by a sudden inability to void. It often presents with suprapubic pain and severe urgency. There is usually a history of preexisting obstructive voiding symptoms related to bladder outlet obstruction or poor detrusor function.

B. **Benign prostatic hyperplasia** is the most common cause of acute urinary retention in men over the age of 50.
   1. Patients present with progressively worsening voiding difficulties, resulting in bladder overdistention and subsequent urinary retention.
   2. Prostate size on digital rectal examination has no bearing on the degree of outlet obstruction because minimal enlargement of the prostate can cause significant obstruction.

C. **Prostate cancer** accounts for 25% of patients with acute urinary retention. Ten percent of patients with prostate cancer initially present with bladder outlet obstruction.

D. **Additional causes of acute urinary retention** include urethral strictures, bladder neck contractures, bladder stones, and acute bacterial prostatitis. Acute urinary retention may be caused by prolonged obstruction, diabetes mellitus, neurologic disorders (spinal cord injury, herniated vertebral disk), and medications.

E. **Urinary retention after surgery** sometimes temporarily develops in elderly men. Preexisting bladder dysfunction or outlet obstruction is usually present.

F. **Anticholinergic medications** (antihistamines, antidiarrheals, antispasmodics, tricyclic antidepressants) can suppress bladder function. Sympathomimetic drugs (decongestants and diet pills) that cause contraction of the bladder neck can precipitate an increase in outlet resistance.

G. **Complications of acute urinary retention** include postobstructive diuresis, bladder mucosal hemorrhage, hypotension, sepsis, renal failure, and autonomic bladder hyporeflexia

H. **Clinical evaluation of acute urinary retention**
   1. Retention is characterized by an inability to void and suprapubic discomfort. A progressive history of difficulty voiding and irritative voiding symptoms, such as frequency, nocturia or urgency is often noted.
   2. Some patients are incontinent as a result of extreme overdistention of the bladder. A past history of gonorrhea, trauma, underlying diseases, or medications should be sought.
   3. Palpate for a distended bladder and assess size and consistency of the prostate. Tenderness of the prostate on rectal examination suggests acute prostatitis; a diffusely hard or nodular prostate suggests carcinoma.
   4. The penis should be examined to rule out phimosis, paraphimosis, or

meatal stenosis. A neurologic exam should include anal sphincter reflex and perineal sensation.

5. **Laboratory evaluation.** Serum electrolytes, blood urea nitrogen (BUN), creatinine, urinalysis, and urine culture.

I. **Management of acute urinary retention**

1. The entire bladder contents should be drained with a Foley catheter. Adequate volume replacement is necessary to prevent hypotension.
2. Lubrication with 2% lidocaine jelly (injected directly into the urethra with a syringe) will facilitate insertion of a urethral catheter. Medium-sized catheters (#18 to #22 French) should be used because they tend to be stiffer and easier to insert than smaller ones.
3. In patients with large prostates, Coude' catheters (which have a curved tip) may be helpful. The curve of the Coude' catheter should be directed superiorly. Other methods of drainage include urethral sounds, filiforms with followers, and percutaneous suprapubic tubes.
4. Admission to the hospital is not required for most patients with acute urinary retention unless infection or renal failure are present. Most patients can be managed with a Foley catheter and discharged home with oral antibiotics and a leg urine bag.

II. Testicular torsion

A. Testicular torsion is an emergency. Delay in treatment may result in testicular loss. A four- to six-hour delay may impair normal testicular function. Torsion can occur at any age; however, it is most common in adolescents, peaking at the age of 15 to 16 years.

B. Testicular torsion presents with sudden onset of pain and swelling in one testicle, occasionally associated with minor trauma. Nausea, vomiting, and lower abdominal or flank pain are common. A history of previous similar episodes with spontaneous resolution is common.

C. A urinalysis is essential in differentiating testicular torsion from epididymitis; however, a negative urinalysis does not rule out epididymitis.

D. **Differential diagnosis of testicular torsion**

1. **Epididymitis** due to Neisseria gonorrhoeae and Chlamydia trachomatis is much more common than torsion in adult men.
2. **Torsion of an appendix testis** or appendix epididymis may mimic testicular torsion. Torsion of the appendix testis may manifest as a tender, pea-sized nodule at the upper pole of the testicle with a small blue-black dot seen through the scrotal skin (the blue dot sign). Management is conservative; however, if there is diagnostic uncertainty, surgical exploration is required.
3. Other less common conditions that may present similarly to torsion include acute hemorrhage into a testicular neoplasm, orchitis, testicular abscess, incarcerated hernia, and testicular rupture.

E. **Physical examination**

1. Testicular torsion usually presents with severe unilateral testicular pain with an acute onset. The pain is associated with an extremely tender testicle with a transverse lie or an anterior epididymis that lies high in the scrotum.
2. With testicular torsion, the testis is usually high in the scrotum (Brunzel's sign). The presence of a cremasteric reflex almost always rules out testicular torsion.
3. Relief of pain by elevation of the affected testis (Prehn's sign) suggests epididymitis. A negative Prehn's sign suggests testicular torsion.

F. **Diagnostic imaging.** Diagnostic testing should not delay surgical exploration in acute torsion. If the diagnosis is unclear, diagnostic tests may be useful. Color Doppler ultrasound is the most valuable diagnostic study, with nearly a 100% sensitivity and specificity.

G. Management of testicular torsion
1. Immediate detorsion is imperative for all cases of testicular torsion. Testicular salvage rates decrease to 50% at 10 hours and to 10-20% at 24 hours.
2. Manual detorsion can be attempted as an urgent measure by rotating the testicle medially about its pedicle. Surgical orchiopexy is still required.
3. If an infarcted testicle is noted during surgical exploration, it should be removed. If the testicle is viable, both testicles should be fixed in the scrotum with nonabsorbable sutures.

III. Priapism
A. Priapism is defined as a prolonged penile erection. Most cases of priapism in adults are idiopathic. In children the most common causes are sickle cell anemia, hematologic neoplasms (leukemia), and trauma.

B. Evaluation of priapism
1. Patients usually complain of a persistent, painful erection. They may have fever and voiding difficulties.
2. Physical examination should include a neurologic evaluation and perineal inspection for neoplasms. Examination of the penis usually reveals a flaccid glans despite a rigid corpora cavernosa. Hematologic studies should be performed to rule out sickle cell anemia and leukemia.

C. Treatment of priapism
1. Early treatment reduces the risk of long-term impotence, which may occur in 50%. Discomfort can be reduced with parenteral narcotic analgesics and sedation. Detumescence may be achieved using cold compresses, ice packs, warm- or cold-water enemas, and prostate massage.
2. If these treatments are unsuccessful, the static blood may be aspirated from the corpora using a large bore needle. Followed by irrigation of the corpora with saline containing a vasoconstricting agent (phenylephrine, epinephrine, or metaraminol).
3. If this process fails to achieve detumescence, a shunt may be created between the affected corpora cavernosa and unaffected corpus spongiosum with a Tru-Cut biopsy needle. When priapism is secondary to sickle cell anemia, therapy also includes hydration, oxygen, and blood transfusion.

References: See page 113.

Vascular and Orthopedic Surgery

Peripheral Arterial Occlusive Disease

Peripheral arterial occlusive disease affects about 18 percent of persons over 70 years of age. The disease presents with intermittent claudication with pain in the calf, thigh or buttock, which is elicited by exertion and relieved with a few minutes of rest. In most cases, the underlying etiology is atherosclerotic disease of the arteries.

I. Pathophysiology
   A. The incidence of claudication rises sharply between ages 50 and 75 years, particularly in persons with coronary artery disease. This condition affects at least 10% of persons over 70 years of age and 2% of those 37-69 years of age.
   B. **Risk factors**. Cigarette smoking is the most important risk factor for PAOD. Seventy to 90% of patients with arterial insufficiency are smokers. Other risk factors include hyperlipidemia, diabetes mellitus, and hypertension.
   C. After five years, 4% of patients with claudication lose a limb and 16% have worsening claudication or limb-threatening ischemia. The five-year mortality rate for patients with claudication is 29%; 60% of deaths result from coronary artery disease, 15% from cerebrovascular disease, and the remainder result from nonatherosclerotic causes.

II. Clinical evaluation of claudication
   A. **Claudication**
      1. The key clinical features of claudication are reproducibility of muscular pain in the thigh or calf after a given level of activity and cessation of pain after a period of rest.
      2. Patients should be asked about the intensity of claudication, its location, and the distance they have to walk before it begins. The degree of functional impairment should be assessed.
      3. **Aortoiliac disease** is manifest by discomfort in the buttock and/or thigh and may result in impotence and reduced femoral pulses. **Leriche's syndrome** occurs when impotence is associated with bilateral hip or thigh claudication.
      4. **Iliofemoral occlusive disease** is characterized by thigh and calf claudication. Pulses are diminished from the groin to the foot.
      5. **Femoropopliteal disease** usually causes calf pain. Patients have normal groin pulses but diminished pulses distally.
      6. **Tibial vessel occlusive disease** may lead to foot claudication, rest pain, non-healing wounds, and gangrene.
      7. **Rest pain** consists of severe pain in the distal portion of foot due to ischemic neuritis. The pain is deep and unremitting, and it is exacerbated by elevation of the foot and is relieved by dangling the foot over the side of the bed.

III. Physical examination
   A. **Evaluation of the peripheral pulses** should include the femoral, popliteal, posterior tibial, and dorsalis pedis arteries. Pallor on elevation of the extremity and rubor when the limb is dependent is common.

Peripheral Arterial Disease

- **B.** Other signs of chronic arterial insufficiency include brittle nails, scaling skin, hair loss on the foot and lower leg, cold feet, cyanosis, and muscle atrophy. The feet should be inspected for skin breakdown or ulceration.
- **C.** Bruits may be auscultated distal to the arterial obstruction. Abdominal examination for a "pulsatile mass" should be performed because of the association between abdominal aortic aneurysm and peripheral arterial disease.
- **D. Ankle-brachial index** is an effective screening tool. The ankle-brachial index is calculated by dividing the ankle pressure by the brachial systolic pressure.
    1. The normal ABI is above 1.0, since the pressure is higher in the ankle than in the arm.
    2. An ABI below 0.9 has a 95 percent sensitivity for detecting angiogram-positive peripheral vascular disease.
    3. An ABI of 0.40 to 0.90 suggests a degree of arterial obstruction often associated with claudication.
    4. An ABI below 0.4 represents advanced ischemia
    5. In patients with an abnormal ankle-brachial index, testing with segmental arterial pressures and a pulse volume recording before and after exercising to the point of absolute claudication are indicated.

Ankle-Brachial Index Interpretation	
Normal	>1
Abnormal	<0.95
Intermittent claudication	0.4-0.9
Severe disease/ischemia	less than 0.4

- **E. Segmental arterial pressures.** The proximal lower extremity pressures should be equal to or greater than the upper extremity pressures, and the drop in Doppler pressure between segments no greater than 20 mm Hg. These studies help predict the location and severity of the disease.
- **F. Arteriography or magnetic resonance angiography** is required to delineate the extent of the disease when intervention is anticipated.

IV. Management

A. Risk factor modification
1. The goals of risk factor modification in patients with PAOD are the same as those in patients with coronary artery disease. Hypertension should be controlled. Beta-blockers do not usually worsen claudication.
2. **Lipid abnormalities** must be treated. The target LDL cholesterol level is less than 100 mg per dL in patients with symptomatic vascular disease.
3. **Tobacco** is directly toxic to the vascular endothelium and worsens atherosclerosis. All patients must abstain from tobacco use.

B. Antiplatelet agents
1. **Aspirin** should be considered for use in any patient with coronary artery disease, cerebrovascular disease or PAOD.
2. **Clopidogrel (Plavix)**, 75 mg qd, or ticlopidine (Ticlid), 250 mg bid with meals, should be considered in patients who are intolerant of aspirin

therapy. Clopidogrel and ticlopidine are platelet inhibitors; however, clopidogrel has a lower risk of neutropenia.

C. **Exercise.** Walking improves the symptoms of claudication. Patients should walk at least three times per week for at least 30 minutes at each session. Near-maximal claudication pain (absolute claudication distance) should be the resting point, and the patient should follow the program for at least six months.

D. **Medication**
   1. **Cilostazol (Pletal)**, 100 mg bid, is a phosphodiesterase inhibitor that suppresses platelet aggregation and acts as a direct arterial vasodilator. Cilostazol results in a 35 percent increase in the distance before claudication and a 41 percent increase in absolute claudication distance.
   2. **Pentoxifylline (Trental)**, 400 mg tid with meals, provides small improvements in the initial claudication distance and absolute claudication distance.

E. **Operative and endovascular procedures**
   1. Most patients with claudication respond to conservative therapy. Surgery is reserved for patients with rest pain or tissue loss. Patients who have intermittent calf claudication alone are not surgical candidates unless the claudication severely limits their lifestyle or occupational functioning.
   2. Patients with rest pain, tissue loss as a result of gangrene, or non-healing ulcers with an ABI less than 0.6 are surgical candidates.
   3. **Percutaneous transluminal angioplasty** has a greater than 90% success rate in the treatment of short-segment aortoiliac occlusive disease, and these results may be improved with the placement of an intra-arterial stent. However, five-year patency rates are only 40-60%.
   4. **Surgical bypass therapy** is an effective treatment for claudication; however, it is associated with 5% morbidity and mortality rates. Aortobifemoral grafting has a 90% 5-year patency rate. Aortoiliac, femoral-femoral crossover, and reversed and in-situ saphenous vein bypass grafting from the common femoral to the popliteal artery have 60-70% 5-year patency rates. A synthetic polytetrafluoroethylene graft (PTFE) is indicated for above knee femoral-popliteal bypass, and it has a 50% 5-year patency rate.
   5. **Axillofemoral bypass** is useful for high risk, elderly patients who are unable to tolerate an aortic procedure.

F. **Management of the acutely threatened limb.** An acutely occluded artery can cause limb loss within hours. The patient will complain of sudden onset of severe unrelenting rest pain. Atrial fibrillation often may cause acute embolic arterial occlusion. These patients require emergency surgical evaluation and immediate heparinization.

Abdominal Aortic Aneurysms

S.E. Wilson, MD

Abdominal aortic aneurysms (AAAs) are the most common type of arterial aneurysm. Approximately 5% of people older than 60 years develop an abdominal aortic aneurysm, and the male-female ratio is 3:1. Other risk factors include smoking, hypertension, and a family history of an aneurysm. Abdominal aortic aneurysms are caused atherosclerosis in 90% of patients; 5% of aneurysms are inflammatory.

I. **Clinical evaluation**
   A. **Abdominal aortic aneurysms** are usually asymptomatic. Aneurysm expansion or rupture may cause severe back, flank, or abdominal pain and shock. Distal embolization, thrombosis, and duodenal or ureteral compression can produce symptoms.
   B. **Physical examination.** Almost all AAAs greater than 5 cm are palpable as a pulsatile mass at or above the umbilicus. Abdominal aortic aneurysms range from 3 to 15 cm in diameter.
II. **Laboratory evaluation.** Complete blood count, electrolytes and creatinine, blood urea nitrogen, coagulation studies, blood type and cross-matching, and urinalysis should be obtained.
III. **Radiologic evaluation**
   A. **Abdominal cross-table lateral films** allow for estimation of aneurysm diameter.
   B. **Ultrasonography and computed tomographic (CT) scanning** demonstrate AAAs with an accuracy of 95% and 100%, respectively.
IV. **Elective management of abdominal aortic aneurysms**
   A. Small aneurysms can be followed using ultrasound or CT scan every 6 months.
   B. Indications for repair include symptomatic aneurysms of any size, aneurysms exceeding 5.0 cm, those increasing in diameter by more than 0.5 cm per year, and saccular aneurysms.
   C. **Preoperative management** includes optimizing cardiopulmonary function and placement of a pulmonary artery catheter or a central venous line. An arterial line permits continuous BP and blood gas monitoring. Two peripheral venous catheters should be placed.
   D. **Operative management.** The aneurysm is approached through a midline abdominal incision and exposed by incising the retroperitoneum.
   E. The duodenum and left renal vein are dissected off the aorta. After heparinization, the aorta is cross-clamped first distal and then proximal to the aneurysm. Aortotomy is then made and extended longitudinally to the aneurysm "neck," where the aorta is either transected or cut in a T fashion. The aneurysm is opened, thrombus is removed, and bleeding lumbar arteries are suture ligated. Using a tube or bifurcation graft, the proximal anastomosis is performed to nonaneurysmal aorta. The distal anastomosis is completed at the aortic bifurcation (tube graft) or at the iliac or femoral arteries (bifurcation graft).
   F. **Endovascular treatment of AAA** uses a catheter to place a stent-graft. Early results suggest an 83% success rate and less than 6% mortality.

References: See page 113.

Orthopedic Fractures and Dislocations

Harry Skinner, MD
Michelle Schultz, MD

I. **Clinical evaluation of the injured limb**
   A. **Physical examination of the injured limb.** 1) Inspection, 2) Palpation, and 3) Movement. Examine the bone for instability and examine the soft

tissue for associated injury. Document neurologic and vascular status.

B. Clinical features of fractures
1. **Pain and tenderness.** All fractures cause pain in the neurologically intact limb.
2. **Loss of function.** Pain and loss of structural integrity of the limb cause loss of function.
3. **Deformity.** Change in length, angulation, rotation and displacement.
4. **Attitude.** The position of the fractured limb is sometimes diagnostic. The patient with a fractured clavicle usually supports the limb and rotates his head to the affected side.
5. **Abnormal mobility and crepitus:** These signs should not be sought deliberately because pain and injury may result.

C. Clinical features of dislocations
1. **A dislocation** occurs when the articular surfaces of a joint are no longer in contact. Subluxation (partial dislocation) is a less severe condition that occurs when the orientation of the surfaces is altered but they remain in contact.
2. **Pain and tenderness.** Severe pain may be completely relieved when the joint is relocated.
3. **Loss of motion.** Both active and passive motion are limited in dislocations.
4. **Loss of normal joint contour.** In the anteriorly dislocated shoulder, the deltoid is flattened and the greater tuberosity of the humerus is no longer lateral to the acromion.
5. **Attitude.** The patient carefully holds the anteriorly dislocated shoulder in abduction and external rotation.
6. **Neurologic injury.** The incidence of neurologic injuries is much higher with dislocations than with fractures. Shoulder dislocations are often associated with axillary nerve injury. Posterior dislocations of the hip can result in sciatic nerve contusion. Careful examination for neurologic status is indicated before any intervention.

II. Clinical description of fractures

A. Anatomic location
1. What bone is fractured?
2. Where on the bone is the fractured?
   a. **Metaphyseal** - at the flare of the bone.
   b. **Diaphyseal** - fracture through the diaphysis (proximal, middle, or distal third of shaft).
   c. **Epiphyseal** - fracture at the end of the bone.
3. Salter classification of fractures (children):
   a. **Type I.** Fracture through physis, between the epiphysis and metaphysis.
   b. **Type II.** Fracture through physis, involving the metaphysis.
   c. **Type III.** Fracture through physis, involving the epiphysis.
   d. **Type IV.** Fracture through physis, involving the metaphysis and epiphysis.
   e. **Type V.** Crush injury to physis, between the epiphysis and metaphysis.

B. Bony deformity:
Describe any change in bone length, angulation, rotation, or displacement.

C. Direction of the fracture line.
Describe the radiographic direction of the fracture.
1. **Transverse** - perpendicular to the long axis of the bone

Orthopedic Fractures and Dislocations

- **2. Oblique** - fracture is at an angle to the bone.
- **3. Spiral** - occurring secondary to torsional stress.
- **D. Comminution:** Fracture with more than two fragments.
- **E. Open vs. Closed:** In an open fracture the bone protrudes through the skin.
- **F. Greenstick Fracture:** one cortex is broken while the other remains intact

III. Radiological evaluation of fractures.
A minimum of two views at right angles to each other should be obtained. Visualize the joint above and below the injury and check for soft tissue swelling. Views of the uninjured extremity are often useful for comparison in children.

IV. Management of fractures
A. Fracture reduction
1. The fracture must be restored to a normal anatomical position
2. Muscle spasm should be relieved with traction, analgesics, and muscle relaxants.
3. Bones must be in apposition, properly aligned in linear and rotatory directions, and set to proper length.
4. Fractures should must be held in place with a splint or cast.

B. Indications for operative treatment
1. Failure of closed methods to reduce or maintain reduction of the fracture.
2. Displaced intraarticular fractures, where the fragments are sufficiently large to allow internal fixation.
3. Multiple injuries - in a multiple trauma patient, operative treatment can allow early mobilization. Early mobilization can sometimes avoid the morbidity and mortality associated with prolonged recumbency.

C. Upper extremity fractures and dislocations
1. **Distal radius fracture** is often associated with fracture of the ulnar styloid. Treatment consists of closed reduction, casting and elevation of the extremity until swelling subsides. After reduction, check alignment with an x-ray, and rule out median nerve injury.
2. **Forearm shaft fracture:** In adults, radius and ulna shaft fractures require open reduction and internal fixation.
3. **Humerus fracture:** X-ray the entire bone and check for radial nerve injury (wrist drop). Humerus fractures are usually treated with a collar and cuff sling or coaptation splint
4. **Clavicle fractures.** Subclavian artery and brachial plexus injury may occur. The fracture should be splinted with a figure of eight bandage or sling. Clavicle fracture rarely requires surgery.
5. **Anterior shoulder dislocation** occurs when the humeral head has been forced anterior to the glenoid. It is usually caused by extension force applied to abducted arm. The patient presents with the arm in slight abduction, and he cannot bring his elbow to the side. There is a slightly depressed deltoid prominence and arm motion causes pain. Axillary nerve injury may occur, causing a sensory deficit over the deltoid. Treatment consists of reduction with gentle traction.
6. **Posterior shoulder dislocation** occurs when the humeral head has been forced posterior to the glenoid. Dislocation may occur secondary to seizures or electrocution. The arm is held in adduction with internal rotation. Treatment consists of reduction with gentle traction.

D. Lower extremity fractures and dislocations
1. **Femoral neck fractures:** Osteoporotic bone predisposes to this intracapsular fracture. Internal fixation or endoprosthesis (artificial hip)

are required.
2. **Intertrochanteric fractures** usually occur in the elderly after a fall. The fracture is located outside the joint capsule. Treatment consists of internal fixation.
3. **Femoral shaft fracture:** Early intramedullary nailing is recommended in adults. This fracture is rarely associated with a fat embolism syndrome.
4. **Patella fracture:** If the bone is nondisplaced, it can be treated in a cast. If it is displaced more than 2 mm, it should be treated with internal fixation. Quadriceps function should be checked.
5. **Tibial shaft fracture** can be treated closed or with internal fixation.
6. **Ankle fracture:** Evaluate the stability of the ankle fracture by examining the joint space between the talus and tibial plafond. Unstable injuries require internal fixation.

E. Knee injuries
  1. Knee ligament testing
     a. **Varus/valgus femur stress test.** The examiner stabilizes the femur, and pressure is exerted outward or inward at the ankle; a tear of the collateral ligament is indicated by excess mobility.
     b. **Anterior drawer test.** Pull tibia anteriorly with the knee flexed 90 degrees to test for tear of anterior cruciate ligament.
     c. **Posterior drawer test.** Push tibia posteriorly with the knee flexed 90 degrees to test for tear of the posterior cruciate ligament.
  2. The most common ligamentous injuries are tearing of the medial collateral ligament by a blow from the lateral side of the knee, and tear of the anterior cruciate ligament by twisting on a planted foot. Brace immobilization is usually sufficient for medial collateral ligament tears.
  3. Dislocation of the knee often results in multiple ligament injury. Popliteal artery trauma should be excluded. Immobilization of the knee, followed by ligament reconstruction should be completed.

Ankle Sprains

A sprain is the most common ankle injury. Injury may range from minor ligamentous damage to complete tear or avulsion. Sprain occurs when stress is applied while the ankle is in an unstable position, causing the ligaments to overstretch. Stresses usually occur during running or walking over uneven surfaces.

I. Clinical evaluation
  A. Ligaments of the lateral ankle consist of the anterior talofibular ligament, calcaneofibular ligament, and posterior talofibular ligament.
  B. Sprains may be classified as first-degree, involving stretching of ligamentous fibers, second-degree, involving a tear of some portion of the ligament with associated pain and swelling, and third-degree, implying complete ligamentous separation.
  C. An inversion injury is the most common type of sprain, causing damage to the lateral ligaments.

II. Physical examination
  A. The examiner's fingertips should be used to check the anterior capsule and medial and lateral ligaments.
  B. **Anterior draw sign** suggests significant injury. The sign is elicited by

grasping the distal tibia in one hand and the calcaneus and heel in the other and sliding the entire foot forward. This is done both with the ankle in neutral position and with 30°° of plantar flexion. With disruption of the anterior or lateral ligaments, 4 mm or more of anterior shift will occur.
   C. **Passive inversion of the ankle** may produce pain. Swelling occurs anterior to the lateral malleolus at the onset; ecchymoses are common. The talus tilts if the calcaneus is adducted.
III. **Radiographic evaluation**
   A. X-rays are useful in cases of moderate to severe injury, helping to identify any associated skeletal injury in addition to assessing degree of ligamentous damage.
   B. A stress view is obtained (with local anesthesia, if necessary) to check for talar tilt. A tilt of more than 15° is suggestive of lateral ligament injury; more than 25°° of tilt is diagnostic.
IV. **Management of ankle sprains**
   A. **Grade I sprains** are defined as stretch of the ligaments without disruption. Grade I sprains should be treated with rest, ice, compression with an elastic bandage, elevation, and weight bearing as tolerated.
   B. **Grade II sprains** consist of partial tears of the ankle ligaments. Grade II sprains should be treated with rest, ice, compression with an elastic bandage, and elevation. A splint can be applied for a few days, followed by early range of motion.
   C. **Grade III sprains** consist of a complete tear of the ligaments. Treatment of grade III strains consists of rest, ice, compression with an elastic bandage, and elevation. A splint or cast can be applied for a short period of time, followed by early range of motion.

References
References may be obtained at www.ccspublishing.com/ccs

Index

Abdominal aortic aneurysm 108
Abdominal wall layers 57
Acetate 25
Aciphex 70
Activated protein C 22
Acute Abdomen 51
Acute Blood Loss 15
Admitting orders 7
Airway Management 45
Albumin 15
American Surgical Association 8
Amikacin 22
Amikin 22
Amino acid solution 25
Aminosyn 25
Ampicillin 21, 87
Ampicillin-sulbactam 87
Ampicillin/Sulbactam 21
Anal fissures 73, 75
Ancef 7, 10
Anectine 45
Angiodysplasia 71
Angiography 72
Ankle sprain 112
Ankle-brachial index 107
Anorectal disorders 74
Anorexia 51
Anterior Nasal Pack 49
Antibiotic preparation for colonic surgery 7
Aortoiliac disease 106
Appendectomy 55
Appendicitis 54
Arterial Line Placement 30
Arterial saturation 46
Arteriovenous malformation 73
ASA 8
Astler-Coller Modification 79
Ativan 47
Autologous blood 16
Axid Pulvules 69
Axillofemoral Bypass 108
Bile 16
Blood 16
Blood Component Therapy 15
Blunt abdominal trauma 34
Breast Cancer 91, 94
Breast cancer screening 91
Breast conservation therapy 95
Breast Cysts 93
Brief operative note 8
Burns 41
Calcium 25
Calculi 102
Carcinoembryonic antigen 78
Cardiac contusions 40
Cardiac tamponade 39
Cefazolin 7, 10
Cefizox 21
Cefotan 7, 10, 21
Cefotaxime 21
Cefotetan 7, 10, 21
Cefoxitin 10, 21, 87
Ceftazidime 21
Ceftizoxime 21
Cefuroxime 21
Central Intravenous Lines 14

Central line 14
Central venous catheter 14
Central Venous Catheterization 27
Chest Tube 14
Chest tube insertion 37
Chief Compliant 5
Chloride 25
Cholecystectomy 87, 89
Cholecystitis 86
Choledocholithiasis 90
Cilostazol 108
Cimetidine 69
Cisatracurium 47
Claforan 21
Claudication 106
Cleocin 22
Clindamycin 22
Clopidogrel 107
Colloid 15
Colonic obstruction 82
Colonic pseudo-obstruction 82
Colonoscopy 72
Colorectal Cancer 77
CoLyte 22
Combined hernia 57
Compazine 10
Constipation 51
Cooper's Ligament 57
Corgard 64
Cranial Nerve Examination 6
Cricothyrotomy 31
Cryoprecipitate 16
Crystalloids 15
CVAT 6
Deep tendon reflexes 6
Demerol 10, 87
Dextrose 24
Diarrhea 16
Diprivan 47
Direct hernias 57
Discharge Note 12
Discharge summary 13
Dislocations 109
Diverticulosis 72
Dobutamine 20
Dobutrex 20
Dopamine 20
Drotrecogin alfa 22
Ectopic pregnancy 55
Electrolyte requirement 25
Electrolytes 6, 16
Endoscopic retrograde cholangiopancreatography 90
Endotracheal Tube 14
Enteral nutrition 23
Epigastric hernias 59
Epinephrine 20
Epistaxis 47
Erythromycin 24
Esomeprazole 62, 70
Esophageal injuries 40
Esophageal varices 63
Eulexin 101
External Hemorrhoids 74
External Inguinal Ring 57

External oblique 57
Famotidine 69
Feeding tubes 14
Femoral Canal 57
Femoral hernias 58
Fentanyl 45
Fever 16
Fibroadenoma 94
First-degree burns 41
Fistula-in-Ano 77
Fistulectomy 77
Fistulotomy 77
Flagyl 22
Flail chest 38
Fluids 16
Flutamide 101
Fortaz 21
Fractures 109
FreAmine 25
Free air 53
Fresh Frozen Plasma 15
Gastric fluid 16
Gastrointestinal Bleeding 61, 70
Gentamicin 22, 87
Glasgow Coma Scale 35
Gleason score 99
GoLYTELY 7, 72
Goodsall's rule 77
Gun shot wounds 33
Head trauma 35
Helicobacter pylori 65
Hematochezia 70
Hemorrhagic gastritis 63
Hemorrhoids 74
HepatAmine 25
Hernia repair 59
Hernias 57
Hespan 15
Hesselbach's Triangle 57
Hetastarch 15
History of Present Illness 5
Hydrocortisone 22
Hydroxyzine 10
Hypertonic saline 15
Iliopsoas sign 53
Imipenem/cilastatin 22
Imodium 24
Impotence 106
Incarcerated hernia 57
Incisional hernias 59
Inderal 64
Indirect Hernia 57, 59
Inflammatory bowel disease 73
Inguinal anatomy 57
Inguinal Hernia 59
Inguinal hernias 57
Inguinal Ligament 57
Inotropin 20
Internal Jugular Vein Cannulation 27
Internal oblique 57
Internal Ring 57
Intestinal Obstruction 81
Intravenous Pyelogram 102
Intropin 20

Intubation 45, 46
Ischemic Colitis 74
Jaundice 52
Kefurox 21
Lactated Ringers 15
Lacunar Ligament 57
Lansoprazole 62, 69, 70
Laparoscopic Cholecystectomy 87
Leriche's syndrome 106
Leuprolide 101
Levator ani syndrome 75
Levophed 20
Lichtenstein repair 60
Linezolid 22, 23
Lipid 23
Lipid solution 24
Locally advanced breast cancer 96
Lomotil 24
Loperamide 24
Lorazepam 47
Lower Gastrointestinal Bleeding 70
Lumbar hernias 59
Lumpectomy 96
Lupron 101
Magnesium 25
Maintenance fluid 16
Mallory-Weiss Syndrome 63
Mannitol 36
Massive hemothorax 38
Mastectomy 96
Mechanical Prep 7
Mefoxin 21, 87
Melena 70
Meperidine 10, 87
Meropenem 22
Merrem 22
Mesenteric Arterial Embolism 80
Mesenteric Arterial Thrombosis 80
Mesenteric Ischemia 80
Metoclopramide 24
Metronidazole 22
Mezlocillin 22
Midazolam 45, 46
Minute ventilation 46
Modified radical mastectomy 96
Morphine sulfate 47
Multiple organ dysfunction syndrome 18
Murphy's sign 17, 53
Nadolol 64
Nafcil 21
Nafcillin 21
Nasal Pack 49
Nasogastric Tubes 14
Needle cricothyrotomy 31
Needle localized biopsy 93
Neo-Synephrine 20
Neomycin 7
Nexium 02, 70
Nimbex 47
Nizatidine 69
Non-protein calories 23
Norcuron 47
Norepinephrine 20
Normal saline 15
Nutritional requirements 23
Obturator hernias 59
Obturator sign 53, 54

Octreotide 64, 86
Ogilvie's syndrome 82
Omeprazole 09, 70
Operative report 8
Oral antibiotic prep 7
Orotracheal Intubation 45
Orthopedics 109
Ovarian cysts 55
Ovarian torsion 55
Packed Red Blood Cells 15
Pancreatic 16
Pancreatitis 83
Pancuronium 47
Pantaloon hernia 57
Pantoprazole 62
Papaverine 81
Past Medical History 5
Pavulon 47
Pepcid 69
Peptic ulcer disease 65
Perianal Abscess 76
Peripheral arterial occlusive disease 106
Peripheral parenteral nutrition 27
Peritoneal lavage 34
Phenylephrine 20
Phosphate 25
Piperacillin 22
Piperacillin/tazobactam 21, 87
Plasmanate 15
Platelets 15
Plavix 107
Pletal 108
Pneumothorax 37
Polyethylene glycol solution 7
Polyethylene glycol-electrolyte solution 72
Post-Operative Management 10
Posterior Pack 50
Postoperative Check 9
Postoperative check 9
Postoperative Fever Workup 16
Postoperative Orders 10
Postural hypotension 61
Potassium 25
PRBCs 15
Prevacid 62, 69, 70
Prevpac 69
Priapism 105
Prilosec 69, 70
Primaxin 22
Procedure Note 12
Prochlorperazine 10

Proctalgia fugax 75
Progress Note 11
Propofol 47
Propranolol 64
Prostate Cancer 97
Prostate specific antigen 97
Protein 23
Protonix 62
Protonix 70
Pruritus Ani 76
Psoas sign 54
Pulmonary artery catheter 14
Pulmonary Artery Catheter Values 29
Pulmonary Artery Catheterization 29
Pulmonary contusions 40
Pulmonology 45
Pulses 6
Purified Protein Fraction 15
Quinupristin/dalfopristin 22
Rabeprazole 70
Radiation therapy 100
Radical prostatectomy 100
Radiographic Evaluation of Common Interventions 14
Radionuclide scan 87
Radionuclide scan or bleeding scan 72
Ranitidine 69
Ranson's criteria 85
Rectus sheath 57
Red Blood Cell Transfusion 15
Reglan 24
Renal Calculi 102
Renal Colic 101
Rest Pain 106
Review of Systems 5
Rovsing's sign 53
Sandostatin 64
Scarpa's fascia 57
Sclerotherapy 65
Sepsis 17, 18, 22
Septic shock 18
Seton Procedure 77
Shock 32
Silver sulfadiazine 44
Sliding hernias 57
Small bowel obstruction 82
Sodium 25
Sphincterotomy 75
Spigelian hernias 59
Sponge Pack 50
Stab wounds 33
Stereotactic core needle biopsy 92
Strangulated hernias 57
Strangulated obstruction 82
Subclavian Vein Cannulation 28
Sublimaze 45
Succinylcholine 45
Surgical Cricothyrotomy 31
Surgical History 5
Surgical physical examination 5
Surgical Progress Note 11
Synercid 22

Systemic inflammatory response syndrome 18
Tagamet 69
Tension pneumothorax 38
Tension-Free Repair 60
Testicular Torsion 104
Tetanus 36
Third-degree burns 42
Thoracic trauma 37
Thoracotomy 37
Ticarcillin 22
Ticarcillin/clavulanate 21, 87
Timentin 21, 87
TIPS 65
Tobramycin 22
Total parental nutrition 24
Tracheostomy 14
Transfusion 15
Transjugular intrahepatic portosystemic shunt 65
Transversalis fascia 57
Transversus abdominous 57
Trauma 32
Traumatic aortic transection 40
Traumatic esophageal injuries 40
Trental 108
Ulcer 65
Umbilical hernias 59
Unasyn 21, 87
Upper Gastrointestinal Bleeding 61
Urinary Retention 103, 104
Urine analysis 6
Urologic Emergencies 103
Vancomycin 22
Vancomycin-resistant enterococcus 22
Variceal bleeding 63
Vascular surgery 106
Vecuronium 47
Venous Cutdown 30
Ventilator Management 46
Versed 45, 46
Vistaril 10
Weaning 47
Whole gut lavage 7
Xigris 22
Zantac 69
Zinacef 21
Zosyn 21, 87
Zyvox 22

Order Form

Current Clinical Strategies books can also be purchased at all medical bookstores

Title	Book	CD
Treatment Guidelines in Medicine, 2004 Edition	$19.95	$36.95
Psychiatry History Taking, Third Edition	$12.95	$28.95
Psychiatry, 2003-2004 Edition	$12.95	$28.95
Pediatric Drug Reference, 2004 Edition	$9.95	$28.95
Anesthesiology, 2004-2005 Edition	$16.95	$28.95
Medicine, 2005 Edition	$16.95	$28.95
Pediatric Treatment Guidelines, 2004 Edition	$19.95	$29.95
Physician's Drug Manual, 2003 Edition	$9.95	$28.95
Surgery, Sixth Edition	$12.95	$28.95
Gynecology and Obstetrics, 2004 Edition	$16.95	$30.95
Pediatrics, 2004 Edition	$12.95	$28.95
Family Medicine, 2004 Edition	$26.95	$46.95
History and Physical Examination in Medicine, Tenth Edition	$14.95	$28.95
Outpatient and Primary Care Medicine, 2005 Edition	$16.95	$28.95
Critical Care Medicine, 2005 Edition	$16.95	$32.95
Handbook of Psychiatric Drugs, 2004 Edition	$12.95	$28.95
Pediatric History and Physical Examination, Fourth Edition	$12.95	$28.95
Current Clinical Strategies CD-ROM Collection for Palm, Pocket PC, Windows, and Macintosh		$49.95

CD-ROMs are compatible with Palm, Pocket PC, Windows and Macintosh.

Quantity	Title	Amount

Order by Phone: 800-331-8227 or 949-348-8404
Fax: 800-965-9420 or 949-348-8405
Internet Orders: http://www.ccspublishing.com/ccs
E-mail Orders: bookorder@ccspublishing.com
Mail Orders:

    Current Clinical Strategies Publishing
    27071 Cabot Road, Suite 126
    Laguna Hills, California 92653

Credit Card Number: _____

Exp: ____/____

A shipping charge of $4.00 will be added to each order

Signature: _____

Check Enclosed _____

Phone Number: (_____)_____

Name and Address (Print):

Admission Orders

- A - admit to
- D - dx
- C - condition
- V - vitals q4h
- A - activity
- A - allergies
- N - nursing — I/Os q4h, neurovascular flap vs Foley to gravity, notify if BP ?
- D - drugs/medications
- D - diet   NPO; soft liquid; ADAT
- D - drains
- I - IVF   D5½ NS w 20 mEQ KCl/L @ 125 cc/hr
- L - Labs / Imaging

Antibiotics

Perioperative ABx

A. Clean procedures — Ancef × 3 doses
  1. immediate preop
  2. intraop
  3. postop

  1 g IV q 8h × 3 doses

B. dirty procedures — Cefotetan
  1 g IV q 12 h × 3 doses

Medications

ABx - Ancef (cefazolin)
  Cefotan (cefotetan)

Pain - Tylenol 3 (acetaminophen/codeine) 1-2 PO q4-6h
  Demerol (meperidine) 50 mg IV q3-4 hr

Stool Softener - Colace 100 mg PO BID

αEmetic - Prochlorperazine (Compazine)
  10 mg IV q4-6hr or suppository q4h

αHistamines -

DVT prophylaxis - Lovenox (enoxaparin)
  SCDS